THE

HEALING

POWER OF

ACUPRESSURE

AND ACUPUNCTURE

THE
HEALING
POWER OF
ACUPRESSURE
AND ACUPUNCTURE

*A Complete Guide to Timeless Traditions
and Modern Practice*

■

M A T T H E W   D .   B A U E R ,   L . A c .

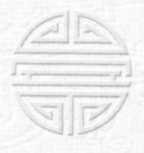

AVERY
A MEMBER OF PENGUIN GROUP (USA) INC.
NEW YORK

Published by the Penguin Group
Penguin Group (USA) Inc., 375 Hudson Street, New York, New York 10014, USA ·
Penguin Group (Canada), 10 Alcorn Avenue, Toronto, Ontario M4V 3B2, Canada (a division
of Pearson Penguin Canada Inc.) · Penguin Books Ltd, 80 Strand, London WC2R 0RL,
England · Penguin Ireland, 25 St Stephen's Green, Dublin 2, Ireland (a division of Penguin
Books Ltd) · Penguin Group (Australia), 250 Camberwell Road, Camberwell, Victoria 3124,
Australia (a division of Pearson Australia Group Pty Ltd) · Penguin Books India Pvt Ltd,
11 Community Centre, Panchsheel Park, New Delhi – 110 017, India · Penguin Group (NZ),
Cnr Airborne and Rosedale Roads, Albany, Auckland 1310, New Zealand (a division of Pearson
New Zealand Ltd) · Penguin Books (South Africa) (Pty) Ltd, 24 Sturdee Avenue, Rosebank,
Johannesburg 2196, South Africa · Penguin Books Ltd, Registered Offices:
80 Strand, London WC2R 0RL, England

Library of Congress Cataloging-in-Publication Data

Bauer, Matthew D.
The healing power of acupressure and acupuncture : a complete guide to
timeless traditions and modern practice / by Matthew D. Bauer.
p.   cm.
Includes bibliographical references and index.
ISBN 1-58333-216-2
1. Acupuncture.   2. Acupressure.   I. Title.
RM184.B38   2004   2004057378
615.8'92—dc22

Printed in the United States of America
10   9   8   7   6   5   4   3   2

This book is printed on acid-free paper. ⊗

Book design by Tanya Maiboroda

I dedicate this to my lovely and loving wife, Gayle: You deserve the dedication in a book of passionate love poems. Unfortunately, my skill as a poet is limited to limericks about men from Nantucket, so I'm afraid this will have to do.

ACKNOWLEDGMENTS

I WANT TO THANK MY PATIENTS, who showed their trust in me by letting me be involved with their care and from whom I learned so much. Whatever else I may do, I am first and foremost a healer, and a healer's blessings are measured by the gratitude of those he serves. Thanks to you, I have been blessed indeed. I also want to thank my family, my wife, Gayle, and my sons Eric and Bryce, for their understanding over the years I worked on this project. I found out something about myself while writing this book: I am not such a nice guy to be around when I am anguishing over exactly how to word my thoughts on a subject I care deeply about. Those closest to me took the brunt of my moods and put up with me anyway. Gayle also caught many mistakes proofreading, and Bryce corrected many of my grammatical errors.

I want to offer a special thanks to three people who were most responsible for making this book possible. Christel Winkler is a wonderful acquisitions editor who wields a light but spot-on scalpel and who took a chance going to bat for a very rough first-time author. Bert P. Krages is a literary agent who likewise took a chance on me and not only did a wonderful job representing me but also gave me extremely savvy advice early on that undoubtedly helped us find a publisher. Claudia Suzanne is an editor, book doctor, and compassionate cheerleader who literally took a cardboard box full of very rough drafts and somehow forged a workable structure for me to begin putting something readable together. Of course, even with the support of these three, I would not have anything to show for my work if the decision-makers at Penguin did not see something worthwhile in this project, for which I am so very grateful. Donna Ikkanda, Jeanine Henderson, and Ron Brown provided me with fine illustrations, and copy editor Martha Ramsey tightened things up nicely.

Some of my colleagues in the healing arts who gave me invaluable feedback include Dr. Elad Schiff, M.D., Dr. Yoon-Hang Kim, M.D., MPH, Ann Bailey, R.N., M.S., L.Ac., Dipl.Ac., and Corinne Axelrod, MPH, L.Ac., Dipl.Ac. I attempted to go to the direct sources whenever possible and was fortunate to get help from key people in the following organizations: Dort Bigg, Executive Director of the Accreditation Commission for the Certification of Acupuncture and Oriental Medicine, Debra Presinger, Interim CEO of the National Commission for the Certification of Acupuncture and Oriental Medicine, C. James Dowden, Executive Director, and Zeus Rivera, MIS Associate of the American Academy of Medical Acupuncture, Dr. John Amaro, D.C., FIAMA, Dipl.Ac. (IAMA) (NCCAOM), L.Ac., of the International Academy of Medical Acupuncture, Barbara Esher, AOBTA CL., Dipl. ABT&Ac. (NCCAOM), L.Ac., Director of Education, American Organization for Bodywork Therapies of Asia,

Dr. David Field, N.D., L.Ac., former President of the California Naturopathic Doctors Association, and Dr. Sally Lamont, ND., L.Ac., former Executive Director of the California Naturopathic Doctors Association. Thank you all for your time and help. I also wish to extend a special thanks to Dr. Zhang-Hee Cho, of the University of California at Irvine, for his immense contributions to the field of acupuncture research as well as for his friendship.

I could not begin to list all of my patients who offered advice and support over the many years I worked on this while I was working on them. Some, though, deserve special mention: the Ross family—Floyd Senior for his clear thinking and introducing me to the work of Joseph Campbell, Floyd Junior for insights on the subject of physics, and especially Kashi Ross for her pointing out that my early attempts to explain the concept of qi were lacking. Others include Allan Andrews, the late Mildred (Billie) Talley, and Mitzi Hiett. I also want to mention the help of a patient, friend, and pioneer in the field of holistic health care information, Suzan Walter, President of the American Holistic Health Association.

I would need an entire book to acknowledge the gratitude I feel toward my foremost teacher, Hua-Ching Ni, a.k.a. Master Ni. I could not imagine anyone else who brings together so many qualities: brilliant insight, truly transcendental spiritualism, humility, humor, an unmatched work ethic, a unique balance of embodying the essence of the ancient with the practical need to stay current . . . the list goes on. As highly as I think of this man, I would be doing a disservice to his teachings if I did not acknowledge that he was trained to pass along the insights derived from those who for thousands of years lived as one with nature, and sought to preserve the lessons they learned. The many insights I learned from Master Ni were made possible because of those who carried this knowledge forward for the benefit of all. My gratitude toward my teacher, then, extends to the countless generations of teachers before him.

CONTENTS

INTRODUCTION

A BLUE-EYED ACUPUNCTURIST

I STICK NEEDLES IN PEOPLE FOR A living. It's okay—I'm an acupuncturist, and that's what we do. Considering that most people hate needles, you might think acupuncturists such as myself would have trouble convincing people to let us stick them, but while this may have been the case fifteen or twenty years ago, today the opposite is true. Not only is my practice quite busy but also the ancient Chinese practice of acupuncture is experiencing an explosion of popularity in virtually every corner of the globe. Clearly, a large number of people have come to believe two things: (1) acupuncture works, and (2) it doesn't hurt.

I had come to those two conclusions myself when I took what most of my friends and family thought to be a bad gamble and enrolled in an acupuncture college in the early 1980s. Back then, the future of acupuncture in the United States was not such a sure thing; in fact, most Americans thought the idea was absurd. "How could poking needles in people help anything?" they would ask.

But those of us who had experienced the effects of acupuncture first-hand knew it worked. Some of us had become fascinated by it and felt a calling to spread the good news to others. Small groups of us found our way to tiny acupuncture schools, many with strange names, and started paying tuition for training in a practice we all knew was a valuable form of treatment, even if we weren't sure it would ever earn us a living.

As difficult as it may be for many to believe, acupuncture has the potential to be an effective form of therapy in virtually every area of medicine. In addition to treating pain, acupuncture is useful for such internal conditions as angina, asthma, bronchitis, constipation, diabetes, and hypertension, as well as disorders involving every organ and gland. Acupuncture also treats skin disorders; reproductive disorders, including infertility, impotence, and most female disorders; neurological disorders, including multiple sclerosis, Parkinson's disease, post-stroke complications, and neuropathy; pediatric, geriatric, and psychiatric disorders; and even such modern problems as chemical dependency and chemical sensitivity, as well as AIDS and its associated complications. A well-trained acupuncturist has the potential to treat a wider variety of patients than virtually any other type of health care professional. Knowing this gave many of the first generations of American acupuncturists the confidence we needed to enter this new-to-the-Western-world field. The problem we faced was that we were the *only* ones who knew this about acupuncture.

BEFORE YOU STICK ME . . .

My first years in practice were both exciting and a struggle. I had settled in a small, conservative community on the eastern border of Los

Angeles County, put out my shingle, and tried to do whatever I could to get patients into my office. Those who found their way to me were often in pretty bad shape. Besides those with common ailments such as back or neck problems, headaches, arthritis, and so on, I saw people with unusual skin, respiratory, internal, and neurological problems. Many were in great pain, and had already tried every type of doctor imaginable without success. Some literally told me in tears that I was their "last hope."

Fortunately, I was able to help most of these people. Slowly, I began to see my first referral patients, many of whom had also tried other, more "conventional" care before seeing me but were somewhat less desperate than those first brave souls who had let this young American acupuncturist treat them. Before proceeding with treatment, the less desperate often wanted to know how acupuncture worked—a reasonable enough request, but one not so easy to accommodate.

Acupuncture is based on the theory that there is an invisible force or energy in nature that the Chinese call *qi* (pronounced "chee," sometimes translated as "chi") and the Japanese call *ki* (key). In a manner similar to blood circulation, qi flows to each cell via a complex network of pathways usually called "channels" or "meridians." If qi gets stuck, it causes an imbalance as upstream cells are flooded with too much qi and downstream cells receive too little. Acupuncture points are those spots where qi has the greatest tendency to get stuck; hence stimulating them with needles (acupuncture) or finger pressure (acupressure) helps free stuck qi and restore normal circulation. Once normal qi circulation is restored, the cells eventually return to their normal, healthy state.

While the foregoing explanation pretty well sums up acupuncture and Chinese medical theory,* I quickly learned it did not suffice for

*I have chosen to use the term "Chinese" instead of "Oriental" medicine because this book focuses on the early roots of these concepts that most authorities agree originated in the region known today as China. I also do this because some object to the word "Oriental" as it was coined in the West. I fully acknowledge and respect the contributions other Far Eastern cultures have made to this healing system.

many of those patients who wanted to understand how acupuncture worked before proceeding with treatment. Some who came for consultations dragged along skeptical spouses who were certain that if acupuncture worked at all, it was only through the power of suggestion. They wanted to know why, if qi is such an important force of nature, modern science has no knowledge of it. If our bodies have a complex network of qi circulation, similar to our vascular system, why has no one ever found the qi channels/meridians, despite countless surgeries and millions of autopsies? And, finally, they demanded an explanation of how the ancient Chinese were able to discover something so elusive that it has evaded modern science.

I spent hundreds of hours explaining the answers to these questions, to the point that I began to look at my patients' education as a sort of personal challenge. I knew in my heart that the theories behind Chinese medicine were every bit as valid as the theories behind modern Western medicine. The difficulty lay in the fact that Chinese medicine is based on concepts born of a different age and culture, not easily translated into modern terms. I took it as a challenge to find explanations of these theories that a rational-thinking modern Westerner could feel comfortable with.

A BOOK IDEA IS BORN

Over time, encouraged by several patients, I became intrigued with the idea of expanding my fifteen- to thirty-minute oral explanations into a book. As I thought about how I would lay out a rational acupuncture explanation in written form, I realized I had a significant problem: since no one knows how acupuncture first began, it's no wonder that Americans tend to be skeptical about the practice. The roots of acupuncture stretch back to prehistoric times, long before the age of recorded history. Along with how the pyramids were built or why Stonehenge was constructed, most historians consider the origin of acupuncture an unsolvable mystery. Yet while Egyptologists attempt to unravel the mystery of the significance of the pyramids and how they may have been built, no one to date has seriously attempted to solve the mystery of how acupuncture came to be.

The more I considered this fact, the more it bothered me. Acupuncture is a product of the same mysterious age that occurred just before the advent of recorded history, when a handful of ancient cultures, known as ancient high civilizations, made incredible advances that baffle us even today. Without realizing what I was getting myself into, I decided I would attempt to address this myself, and began what would turn into a ten-year labor of love.

I felt my training would help me address this mystery. Several years before my formal acupuncture schooling, I had begun studying ancient Taoist (pronounced "dowist") philosophy with one of the world's leading authorities on Taoism, the oldest philosophic system of the Chinese people. Hua-Ching Ni, affectionately known to his students as Master Ni, had been trained since childhood to pass along the ancient teachings of his tradition, and had moved to the United States in 1976 to teach Taoist science, philosophy, and spirituality and to work as a healer. Over the next twenty-five years, Master Ni published more than forty books on a wide variety of Taoist subjects. While none of these books specifically dealt with the question of acupuncture's roots, it occurred to me that some of the ancient teachings contained in these works offered clues that could shed some light on this mystery.

I became fascinated with ancient Taoist folk history, and I acquired a respect for the logic of Taoist science. More important, the spiritual aspects of Taoism struck a chord deep within me and changed my life forever. I didn't simply learn about Taoism; I became a Taoist. My experience treating my patients with acupressure and acupuncture, as well as my growth as a practicing Taoist, helped me to pursue the question of how this healing system may have begun. I say *may* have begun because, as with the pyramids, it is unlikely this mystery will ever be solved once and for all. It is my hope, however, that exploring the roots of this healing system may help those unfamiliar with it to better understand it and that this will encourage them to take advantage of it. I also hope to encourage more Eastern and Western specialists to explore this subject. I hope this because I am convinced that the more we learn about the roots of acupuncture and acupressure, the better we will understand how to help ease pain and suffering today and in the future.

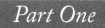

Part One

EXPLAINING

THE

UNEXPLAINABLE

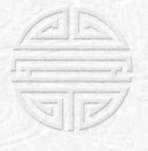

Chapter One

A SPIRITED SCIENCE

Oh, East is East, and West is West, and never the twain shall meet,
Till Earth and Sky stand presently at God's great Judgment Seat.
—RUDYARD KIPLING, "The Ballad of East and West"

W HEN I FIRST BEGAN MY STUDIES of Taoism, I came face-to-face with a manner of thinking every bit as sure of itself as modern Western thought, yet so different that I readily understood why Kipling was sure "never the twain shall meet." Like everyone I'd ever known, I had spent my life accepting the concept that doctors took care of our bodies by ordering x-rays and lab tests, prescribing drugs, and performing surgery, while religions dealt with matters of the spirit. Countless lives were saved every day thanks to the great advancements medical science had made since evolving from such barbaric earlier practices as applying leeches or bleeding patients. Medicine was always making progress, augmenting its set of rules and procedures with hard, replicable, scientific facts. Who knew what miracles future doctors might discover in their laboratories? One thing was certain, though: the rigors of modern science left no room for such unproven quackery as acupuncture and acupressure.

After studying Taoism, I learned to appreciate Chinese medicine and Taoist philosophy but felt out of step with my own culture's reliance on Western science. Today, thanks to researchers such as Zang-Hee Cho, professor of radiological sciences and psychiatry at the University of California, Irvine (UCI), one of the world's foremost authorities on medical imaging technologies, we finally have objective scientific proof that, rather than chicanery or fraud, acupuncture is a legitimate form of therapy that causes changes in the brain and ultimately, body chemistry.

Using functional magnetic resonance imaging (fMRI), an imaging technology he helped pioneer, Dr. Cho can measure the oxygen consumption of brain cells, indicating the degree of activity of these cells. As a result, researchers can actually "see" the brain in action. When a light is shined in a subject's eyes, for example, fMRI records the sudden increased activity in the visual cortex at the back of the brain.

In his very first acupuncture study carried out in 1997, Dr. Cho's research team shined a light in twelve subjects' eyes and measured the predictable activation in their brains' visual cortexes. He then had an acupuncturist needle them at a point on their little toe (Bl67) known for some two thousand years to be effective in treating various vision problems. The result astonished him: four of the twelve subjects showed increases in their visual cortexes similar to having a light shined in their eyes, while eight showed a marked decrease in activity! As happens with many surprising scientific discoveries, Dr. Cho at first thought there was some sort of problem with the way the computerized data had been processed, but after rechecking all the data he found the results were accurate. Befuddled by the results, he discussed them with one of the acupuncturists on his research team, who told Dr. Cho he believed he knew why some subjects showed increases while others showed decreases in activity: it was the yin/yang effect.

As I will show in following chapters, the concept of yin and yang is one of the most important foundations of Chinese science in general and Chinese medicine in particular. Yin energy is considered passive or inactive, while yang energy is considered active. Acupuncturists have long claimed that acupuncture helps the body to adjust itself, increasing what is underactive and decreasing what is overactive. Dr. Cho's researcher went so far as to claim that he could predict which of the twelve subjects' visual cortexes showed increased activity and which showed a decrease by performing a Chinese medicine diagnosis that classifies a person as yin or yang. The yin, or underactive, person should show an increase in activity after receiving acupuncture, while the yang, or overactive subject should show a decrease. After performing this type of diagnosis (explained in chapter 2), and with no knowledge of which subject had which fMRI result, he correctly guessed eleven out of twelve results! Finally, the same twelve subjects had acupuncture on another toe, one not known to have any effect on vision problems. This showed no changes in their visual cortexes.

Professor Cho did several other studies—some of which have been duplicated by other researchers—demonstrating the correlation between acupuncture points traditionally known to treat specific problems and the regions of the brain controlling those parts of the body. His studies offer convincing proof to even the skeptical Western scientific mind of acupuncture's ability to cause real physiologic changes—something Chinese science has understood since ancient times. In fact, in stark contrast to the evolution of Western medicine over hundreds of years, the foundation of Chinese medicine is much the same today as it has been for thousands of years—rooted in a profound ho-

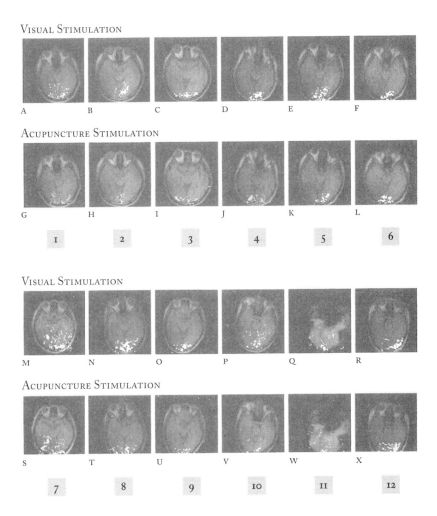

These twelve subjects had a light shined in their eyes (visual stimulation), causing increased activity in their visual cortex (boxes A–F and M–R).

When the same twelve subjects had an acupuncture point on their little toe stimulated (acupuncture stimulation) the first four showed a decrease in their visual cortex activity (boxes G–J), while the next eight showed an increase (boxes K–L and S–X).

listic science developed by the ancient Taoists and based on the mysterious, metaphysical concepts of qi and yin/yang. These concepts, which eventually spread throughout the Far East, formed the very foundation of Chinese culture and helped make China one of the world's most advanced civilizations for more than three thousand years, up until the scientific and industrial revolutions of the nineteenth century sparked great advancements in the West.

Much of what we now understand about the technological achievements of China's advanced civilization—the great cities, with buildings, bridges, and waterways far beyond the scale of anything Marco Polo had ever witnessed back in thirteenth-century Europe; the concepts of burning rocks (coal) and planting crops in rows; the compass, the decimal system, masts and rudders of sailing ships, gunpowder, paper, the printing press—can be credited to Joseph Needham and his Cambridge University research team. In his extensive series of texts on the history of Chinese science, *Science and Civilization in China*, Dr. Needham details many key advancements credited to Western origins that had actually originated in China hundreds or even thousands of years before they appeared in the West. While reporting all these marvels, however, neither he nor Marco Polo before him touched on the reason the ancient Chinese were able to realize these great advancements: their key scientific laws, grounded in observation of nature and discovered in prehistoric time. It was these principles that also led their doctors to treat diseases of the body, mind, and spirit with acupuncture, acupressure, and Chinese herbs.

It took several years for me to comprehend the fundamental difference between modern Western and Chinese science. I finally concluded that the single most important difference between Chinese and Western science is their views of spirituality.

A TALE OF TWO SCIENCES

The great seventeenth-century scientist Galileo is often referred to as the "father" of Western science, in part because he started the idea of using experiments to prove the validity of scientific theories rather than relying on logic alone, as had been done since the days of Aristotle. Galileo also played a pivotal role in a turning point in the history of Western science after he published a book supporting the Copernican theory that the sun, not the earth, was the center of our system of planets, or solar system. The Catholic Church believed such theories contradicted holy scripture, and they threatened to excommunicate the aging Galileo, a devout Catholic, unless he recanted his support of the Copernican theory. Even after Galileo recanted his support, he was forced to spend his last days under virtual house arrest.

Although the Catholic Church hoped to make an example of Galileo, doing so did not solve their problem. New inventions, such as the telescope, together with the scientific method of experimentation, were beginning to uncover facts both impossible to dispute and at odds with the Church's ideas. It came to seem unlikely they would be able to stem the tide of new discoveries as they had done with Galileo. Over time, scientists and the Church worked out a compromise of sorts. Science would be free to investigate the realm of the physical universe without interference from the Church, provided the realm of spirituality remained solely within the Church's authority. Western science went on to become the dominant authority on matters of the physical universe, but, remaining true to the theology vs. science compromise, has never seriously turned its attention to investigate questions of spirituality. Whenever questions of spirituality are posed to scientists, they commonly respond that such matters are not within the "realm" of science, as they are matters of "faith."

CHINESE SCIENCE

Chinese science, in contrast, did not evolve with any such compromise. The ancient Chinese, like people all over the world going back tens of thousands of years, were very interested in matters of spirituality as well as matters of the physical universe. Hence the ancient Taoists' search for truth included both the physical and spiritual realms, with the result that Chinese science developed different laws from those in the West. They even created a symbol for their unique scientific system to demonstrate the inclusion of both the physical and spiritual natures of the world (see the illustration below).

What is known to many as the "yin/yang" symbol is really a kind of formula or symbolic equation that represents the most important laws of Chinese science. One such law, unique to Chinese science, is the *law of opposites*, which declares that everything, in all of creation, must have an opposite. Nothing can exist alone; all phenomena come in pairs of opposites. Hence half the yin/yang symbol is white, and half is black. Another law: not only is everything paired with an opposite, everything contains at least some of its opposite partner within itself, represented by the little white circle within the back half and the little black circle within the white half.

According to oral folk history, the law of opposites was inspired by the observations by the ancient Chinese that all nature seems to come

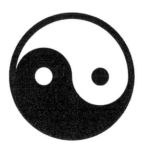

in pairs. For instance, there are two genders: male and female. People use two legs to walk, and birds use two wings to fly. Each day is divided into day and night, dominated by the sun and moon, respectively. Left and right, hot and cold, creation and destruction, inhalation and exhalation, and so forth: the ancient Chinese observed countless examples of pairs of yin/yang opposites.

While some might scoff at the idea of these examples constituting proof of a scientific law, Western science has itself been proving that law correct with its own recent discoveries. According to Western science, all material objects are composed of differing arrangements of the smallest possible building blocks, atoms, which were first detected in the early twentieth century. It was soon discovered however, that atoms were not the smallest possible things but where themselves made up of smaller components—the three subatomic particles, consisting of the positively charged proton and neutral neutron, forming the nucleus, and the negatively charged electron that orbits the nucleus. Later, it was discovered that even these subatomic particles were made of smaller components, called quarks. Chinese science, however, does not allow for a "smallest possible" object because the divisions of yin/yang carry into infinity.

FACTORING IN SPIRIT

The realm of spirituality is also represented in the yin/yang symbol, owing to the fact that the law of opposites was seen as holding true across all scales or levels of reality. On a small scale, the yin/yang symbol represents the relationship between tiny things, like positive and negative subatomic particles. On a bigger scale, it denotes the relationship between paired phenomena such as male and female genders, or the sun and the moon. On the largest scale, it expresses the relationship between the entire physical realm and its logical opposite, the spiritual realm. Thus, a single law that predicts every known fact of our physical universe also predicts that an opposite reality—that of spirituality—must coexist with the physical realm. Like the black and white halves of the yin/yang symbol, the two opposite realms of spirit and matter *together* make up the whole of reality. The idea of separating these two as we have done in the West probably never even occurred to the ancient Chinese.

When I would explain all this to my patients or in group talks, I would encounter two distinct responses: some people would nod and be impressed that the ancient Chinese had come up with such a simple theory that explains so much, while the skeptics would point out I was talking philosophy, not science. The logical conclusion I presented—that the validity of law of opposites for things in the physical realm proves the coexistence of a spiritual realm—was just a theory with no proof, they would say. And they were correct, insofar as what I have described so far about the relationship between the material and spiritual realms is more philosophy than science. But the fault lies not with the law but with my simplified explanation for the sake of brevity. You see, long before Galileo, the ancient Taoists had pioneered the concept of conducting experiments to validate their theories, including the law of opposites.

The types of experiments the ancient Taoists carried out and duplicated over many successive generations differ by necessity from those conducted in Western science, because the experiments utilized in Western science were designed only for testing theories dealing with the physical realm. Testing the spiritual realm requires experimentation with a different version of the scientific method. To understand the Taoist scientific method, however, requires an introduction to a concept absolutely essential to Chinese science, also represented in the yin/yang symbol: the concept of qi.

BETWEEN THE TWO

In addition to symbolizing the law of opposites by virtue of the black and white halves, the yin/yang symbol shows the two halves integrated as one, thus indicating not only the duality of yin and yang but the trinity of yin and yang *and* their integration as one whole. In Taoist numerology, the yin/yang symbol is represented by the number 3 and is sometimes called a *three-in-one*. The third, integrating factor, which harmonizes yin and yang and serves as a bridge between the two, is considered neutral; that is, neither yin nor yang. The concept of a mysterious middle ground between two opposites is very common in traditional Chinese culture. The original name for China itself was the "Middle Kingdom" or "Central Territory," referring to the mystic realm "Between Heaven and Earth." Hence the third, integrating factor that bridges the material and spiritual realms is qi, the mysterious force of nature that is the unique cornerstone of Chinese science.

The concept of qi has no equal in Western science because Western science, evolving as it did under a policy of noninvolvement with matters of spirituality, is unequipped to address the subject, much less detect the reality, of a force that integrates the physical and spiritual realms.* The experiments carried out by the ancient Taoists to explore and confirm the spiritual realm were based on qi, especially the qi of the person doing the experiment. This, again, contrasts with the Western scientific method, which dictates that the person carrying out the experiment must remain an uninvolved observer. In the Taoist scientific method, the person carrying out the experiment is far from unin-

---

*Because Western culture has always completely separated physical and spiritual matters, no term was ever coined to describe a force that bridges the two; *energy*, or *subtle* or *vital energy*, is as close as anyone has ever come. These words only confuse people, however, because they make people think that qi is some kind of energy as understood in Western science terms, which is not correct. Even the Western concept of "vitalism," traced to early Greek thought, does not capture the essence of the term *qi*.

volved as they become, in essence, the laboratory in which the experiment is carried out.

Like everything else in creation, humans are a three-in-one of physical matter, spirit, and qi. Qi bridges an individual's physical and spiritual elements, just as it does the physical and spiritual realms as a whole.

By focusing on balancing one's qi, one can develop the ability to synchronize oneself with the balanced qi of nature. Because the qi of nature bridges the physical and spiritual realms, the more one's qi becomes synchronized with the qi of nature, the more one can bridge these two realms and experience the realm of spirit firsthand.

Think of it this way: the relationship between yin and yang is like the two sides of a seesaw. When one side goes up, the other goes down, and vice versa. Between the two sides is a balancing point, or fulcrum. If the balancing point is closer to one side, the seesaw will be inclined to tilt to that side. If the balance point is perfectly balanced between the two, it encourages the two sides to find their true balance.

The ancient Taoists believed we human beings once had a good balance between our spiritual and physical sides, but over many thousands of years of evolution, we overemphasized the physical. As the physical focus rose, the spiritual focus declined, and the balance point, or qi, between yin (physical) and yang (spiritual) became slanted toward the physical side. Hence people shifted toward the physical and lost touch with their spiritual nature. The early Taoists developed methods to counter this tendency by balancing an individual's qi. They encouraged students to practice these methods so they could confirm the existence of their spiritual nature for themselves rather than rely on religious faith or even philosophical logic. By eating a carefully balanced diet, taking certain herbs, performing special exercises such as tai chi chuan or qi-gong, avoiding overindulgence in sexual activity, and doing specialized meditative practices, an individual can restore the balance between their physical and spiritual natures. These practices also have the added benefit of helping to restore and preserve one's health.

People who successfully practice these methods often undergo a profound shift in their perception of reality. Some will not only have their health improve, they will have mystical experiences, especially during meditations, in which they literally encounter the spiritual realm. I say this because I have practiced some of these methods and have had similar experiences myself. It was having this type of firsthand experience, rather than faith in an ultimate power or trust in the philosophy I studied, that convinced me the ancient Taoists were correct to assert there is another layer of reality available for us to study (and enjoy).

Skeptics will say that none of what I've described about connecting with the spiritual realm qualifies as science because these examples are merely individual experiences, possibly even delusions. It is very hard for the Western mind, trained to trust only a certain type of "proof," to accept the validity of self-centered experiments. But what if the ancient Taoists were right? What if the scientific method of proof through experimentation could be applied to spirituality, but only through individual "inner" exploration? What if the Western scientific method, admittedly impotent in matters of spirituality, needs to undergo changes in order that we may finally bring the rational perspective of science to the study of matters of the spirit?

Chapter Two

CHINESE HEALTH SCIENCE

T HE OLDEST KNOWN BOOK TO DE-
scribe Chinese science in detail, the *Yellow Emperor's Classic of Medicine*, is framed as a series of discussions between one of the most
important figures in Chinese culture, the Yellow Emperor, and his top
court physicians. Known as the "father" of the Chinese people, the Yellow Emperor reigned from 2696 to 2597 BCE and is credited, in addition to his contributions to Chinese medicine, with developing or
helping to develop the calendar, the compass, silk, and systems of astronomy and numerology. Scholars tend to be skeptical about the legends attributed to this great figure; nevertheless, most of them agree
that the *Yellow Emperor's Classic* dates back to at least two hundred
years BCE and is the oldest known book to discuss the principle element of Chinese health science, acupuncture.

The *Yellow Emperor's Classic* is divided into two sections. The first, the *Suwen,* or "Basic Questions," spells out the holistic basis of Chinese science, while the second, the *Lingshu,* or "Mystical Pivot," goes into more detail about specific acupuncture techniques.

The *Suwen* describes the essence of Chinese science as it relates to health and disease, portraying the individual human as a "three-in-one" of matter, spirit, and qi, whose various parts (organs, glands, senses and so forth) are themselves composed of smaller units of matter, spirit, and qi. Just as every individual is made up of many parts, he or she is also part of the surrounding environment, which is likewise composed of matter, spirit, and qi. Both the external and our internal environments are in a state of continual change, which in turn creates a constant need to balance or harmonize our internal environment with the external environment. Internal-environment imbalances create disorder or disease; restoring balance with acupuncture or other techniques restores health.

When the *Yellow Emperor's Classic* discusses this need to restore balance between one's ever-changing internal environment and the ever-changing external environment, it underscores another fundamental law of Chinese science: everything in nature is in a state of continual change. Like the law of opposites, the "law of continual change" is also represented in the yin/yang symbol, which was designed to illustrate constant cyclic motion. The "head" of the white half is pushing itself forward, attracted to the "tail" of the black half while being repulsed by its own "tail." The same is true for the black half. According to Chinese science, the attraction of opposite-polarity forces (yin/yang) and the repulsion of like-polarity forces (yin/yin or yang/yang) fuels the constant evolution of all creation. (For a list of the most important traditional laws of yin/yang, see appendix A.) The ancients explored the law of continual change in the oldest known book in Chinese culture, the *I-Ching,* or *Book of Changes,* a collection of eight symbols thought to be perhaps six thousand to ten thousand years old.

A Different Evolution

Chinese science's view that everything in Creation is in a state of constant evolution is quite different from what Western science has believed throughout most of its history, thus explaining once again why Chinese and Western sciences took very different paths, especially in their methods of measuring nature. One common goal Chinese and modern Western science share is their attempt to place the vast and complex natural world into a perspective the human mind can both understand and communicate to others. This requires standardized methods for measuring what is being observed. Simply put, measuring is crucial to all sciences, and having a reliable "yardstick," so to speak, is crucial to the act of measuring. This is true whether measuring mass with the yardstick of tons or grams, time with the yardstick of centuries or seconds, or space with the yardstick of kilometers or yards, and so on.

Western science established measuring systems with the belief the yardsticks it employed were stable, or unchanging. Time and again, however, Western science has had to find new yardsticks as the old ones were found to be variable. The motion of the sun, moon, and planets were once measured from what was thought to be a stable earth. The idea of a moving earth was revolutionary because it greatly complicated the process for measuring everything moving around it. Albert Einstein is considered such a great genius because he single-handedly figured out that the yardstick of time was unstable, or "relative." According to Einstein, the only constant in nature we can rely on as a stable yardstick is the speed of light, although even this has recently been questioned.

Chinese science, on the other hand, developed with the concept that everything changes; therefore, the fixed mathematical formulas so relied on in Western science were not used to try to understand nature. The Chinese did use numbers—the *Yellow Emperor's Classic* is full of numerological references—but they did not consider those numbers to be absolutely fixed.

As Western science has continually rethought its measuring systems, a newer version of Western science has begun to emerge that utilizes principles very similar to those in Chinese science. Cutting-edge modern theories such as string theory, chaos theory, systems thinking, and cybernetics; models such as "self-organization"; and principles such as the uncertainty principle come much closer than anything in the Western past to Chinese science's laws of a constantly evolving, holistically interconnected universe.

DEALING WITH CHANGE

How did Chinese science deal with the idea that nothing is static, that all is in a state of change? How could they measure anything if they believed that all yardsticks must flucuate? Behind the continual change of all creation, the ancient Chinese saw something that did not change—a pattern. As things evolve, they rise, peak, and then decline. Some things may rise, peak, and decline quickly, like a mushroom or a housefly, whose life only spans a few days. Other things rise, peak, and decline more slowly, like a mountain taking millions of years to spring forth from the bowels of the earth and then erode or a bristlecone pine tree spanning thousands of years between emerging as a tiny sprout and then returning to the soil. No matter how relatively long or short a time span, all things continually rise, peak, and decline. The rising is yang, the declining is yin, and the peaking is the middle/transitional ground between the two.

And this is the "yardstick" Chinese science uses: the three-in-one of rising, peaking, and declining. At some point, the ancient Chinese expanded on this concept and divided the rising phase and declining phases into two phases. Under this more detailed version, the evolution of all things was divided into five phases: (1) the birth of rising, or "young yang"; (2) the maturity of rising, or "mature yang"; (3) the transition from rising to declining (neither yin nor yang); (4) the birth of declining, or "young yin"; and (5) the maturity of declining, or "mature yin." This "five phases of evolution" system became the most popular system of measurement in Chinese science.

A good way to understand the five phases of evolution is by relating it to the four seasons. A complete rotation through all five phases is like a complete rotation of the earth around the sun; as the earth rotates, the climate changes. The concept of dividing a year into four seasons, like cutting a pie into four equal slices, was invented during the age of the ancient high civilizations to help people of that age better grasp the complexity of climate variations so they might benefit from this knowledge, especially in agriculture. The ancient Chinese used the same system for dividing the cyclic evolution of all in nature, with the middle, transitional phase—sometimes referred to in America as "Indian summer"—counted as a fifth slice by some, representing the point at which rising (yang) transitions into declining (yin).

By dividing the rotation of evolution in the same manner, the ancient Chinese could study a single slice or phase at a time, while also pondering how each slice affects and is affected by the other slices, in true "holistic" fashion. Just has we have come to recognize that each season has its own essential characteristics, the Chinese ascribed specific characteristics to each of the five phases, and focused their study on understanding how the characteristics inherent within each phase dynamically interacted within the whole.

THE FIVE PHASES IN MEDICINE

The *Yellow Emperor's Classic* details how the concept of the five phases of evolution applies to matters of health and disease and reveals how

FIVE PHASES OF EVOLUTION TABLE		
	1. Young Yang	**2. Mature Yang**
Season	Spring	Summer
Organs	Liver, gallbladder	Heart, small intestine
Sense	Sight	Taste
Taste	Sour	Bitter
Color	Green	Red
Emotion	Anger	Joy
Vocal manifestation	Shouting	Laughter
Physical manifestation	Muscles/tendons	Vessels
Physical essence	Saliva	Marrow
Physical action	Twitching	Itching
Climate	Wind	Heat
Element	Wood	Fire
Planet	Jupiter	Mars

that system was used to measure or classify things in the field of medicine. Each season, for example, was classified as relating to one of the five phases in regard to the health effects of the ever-changing external environment.

Thus, if an individual tends to have too much "mature yang" (second) phase qi in his or her internal environment, for example, the symptoms of this "imbalance" will worsen in the summer, due to a preponderance of the same qi in the external environment during that season. Conversely, his or her symptoms will improve during winter,

3. Transition: Neither Yin nor Yang	4. Young Yin	5. Mature Yin
Between summer & autumn	Autumn	Winter
Spleen/pancreas, stomach	Lungs, large intestine	Kidneys, bladder
Touch	Smell	Hearing
Sweet	Hot-pungent	Salty
Yellow	White	Black
Pensive	Sadness	Fear
Singing	Crying	Groaning
Flesh	Skin	Bone
Vital essence	Blood	Sexual essence
Hiccuping	Crying	Shivering
Humidity	Dryness	Cold
Earth	Metal	Water
Saturn	Venus	Mercury

the "mature yin" (fifth) phase, as the prevailing qi of the external environment will be the exact opposite and thus will tend to balance out the individual's internal imbalance.

The *Yellow Emperor's Classic* also divided the internal environment into five categories. Each of the five senses relates to one of the five phases, as do the five "major" organs. Different bodily tissues, secretions, and emotions were likewise categorized as relating to one of the five phases. Note in this chart that each phase is associated with a particular "element" illustrating its essential qualities and characteristics.

Because of this popular association, the "five phases of evolution" became known to most as the "five elements."

QI IS THE KEY

Perhaps the most confusing aspect of Chinese medicine is how the ancient Chinese viewed the relationship between the physical components of the body, especially the organs, and qi. The best analogy I have found over the years to help explain this is to consider the relationship between an object and its shadow.

In the presence of light and a suitable background, a three-dimensional object casts a two-dimensional shadow. While object and shadow are not one and the same, a dependent relationship exists between them. The shape of the lower-dimensional shadow is determined by the shape of the higher-dimensional object. The ancient Chinese believed the realm of eternal spirit to be more fundamental than the temporal, three-dimensional, material realm. As qi is the bridge between material and spiritual, the relationship of qi and the material realm is similar to that between an object and its shadow, with qi being akin to the higher-dimensional object and all material things (such as organs) being akin to the lower-dimensional shadow. In other words, everything in the material realm is determined by the status of qi because the status of qi is determined by the status of the most essential spirit. Qi is elusive but less so than the most elusive spirit.

DIAGNOSIS

While recognizing that the internal organs and glands are critical to the health of the physical body, the ancient Chinese viewed the organs as the physical manifestations of the body's core qi. The practice of

Chinese medicine, therefore, involves two primary tasks: assessing a patient's core qi, as measured against the yardstick of the five phases of evolution, and then restoring qi balance with acupuncture or other methods. Qi cannot be seen, felt, tasted, heard, or smelled any more than a shadow can appreciate the third dimension of depth, so assessing qi imbalances is not easy for those humans who have lost touch with their spiritual nature and whose perception is consequently limited to the lower-dimensional material realm. Nevertheless, using the five senses, a practitioner can approximate the qualities of qi, just as one can surmise some features of an object by studying its shadow. The ancient Chinese developed many methods to determine the state of an individual's qi by utilizing the five senses to study different aspects of that person. Of these many diagnostic methods, the two that became most popular among doctors of Chinese medicine are pulse and tongue diagnosis.

Chinese tongue diagnosis involves making several observations about the tongue's shape, color, and texture, including details of any coating. Chinese pulse diagnosis involves feeling for very intricate characteristics of pulse size, shape, and tone, as well as rate. A bright red tongue with a yellow coating and a thin, rapid pulse, for example, indicate excess heat inside the body, while a pale tongue with a white coat and a slow pulse indicate too much internal cold. According to Chinese "holistic" theory, every part of the body is connected to the whole body, just as every part of the universe is connected to the whole universe. Every part both affects and is affected by every other part. Consequently, the status of the whole is reflected in every part, just as any piece of a hologram can convey the image of the entire hologram. The ability to learn the status of the whole from the study of any part is limited only by the individual's skill in deciphering the impressions that the whole leaves on the parts.

The ancient Chinese wanted to understand what was going on inside the body, especially the qi connected with the internal organs and glands. These "parts" could not be directly observed without causing undue damage: you can't cut open the abdomen to see what the stomach looks like without doing more harm than good. In theory, one could learn information about the qi associated with the stomach or other internal organs by observing any part of the body—the eyes, hair, fingernails, and so on—so the Chinese developed diagnostic methods based on those and other parts of the body. Tongue and pulse diagnosis most likely became favored because they are a part of the "inside" that *can* be observed from outside without causing harm. In other words, the tongue and pulse represent a middle ground (bridge) between the inside and outside of the body—yet another example of the Chinese science tendency to focus on the pivotal middle between yin (inside) and yang (outside).

How the Chinese deciphered the impressions the whole body makes on the tongue and pulses follows the concepts of three-in-one and the closely associated five phases of evolution. The body's internal organs were grouped into three sections. The upper section, from the base of the throat to the diaphragm, houses the heart and lungs. The middle section, from the diaphragm to the navel, houses the digestive organs, including the stomach, liver, gallbladder, and what is translated as the spleen, although many authorities think the Chinese were referring to the pancreas. The lower section, from the navel to the pubic region, represents the reproductive and elimination organs, including the kidneys, bladder, and intestines. Both tongue and pulse diagnosis follow this model also. The base of the tongue relates to the lower section (reproductive and elimination qi), the middle of the tongue to the middle region (digestive qi), and the tip of the tongue to the upper region (circulation/respiration qi).

By observing the tongue, information can be gathered about the conditions inside the body. A bright red tip, for example, indicates excess heat in the upper region of the heart and/or lungs. A thick, greasy coating in the middle of the tongue indicates an accumulation of thickened moisture in the middle, digestive region.

While pulses in different areas of the body were sometimes felt, the most common pulse used in Chinese diagnosis is the radial found at both wrists near the base of the thumb. This pulse is felt with three fingers—index, middle, and ring—with the index finger placed at the wrist crease, the middle finger just above the index (moving up from the wrist toward the elbow), and the ring finger placed just above the middle finger. The index finger feels for the upper region of the body, the middle finger for the middle region, and the ring finger for the lower region. A weak pulse felt with the middle finger indicates a weakness in the digestive system. A rapid, thin pulse under the ring finger indicates that heat has consumed yin qi of the reproductive system.

Both tongue and pulse diagnosis involve a myriad of complex details, too involved to go into here. Pulse diagnosis is especially complex, as there are at least twenty-eight different pulses that may be felt, and the skill needed to distinguish each is equal to the skill needed to master a delicate stringed musical instrument. It takes training and experience to understand the subtle signs or clues these diagnostic meth-

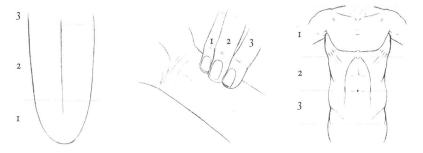

In these drawings, the tip of the tongue and section of the radial artery felt under the index finger (1) relate to the upper region of the torso, the middle of the tongue and artery section under the middle finger (2) relate to the middle of the torso, and the base of the tongue and artery section under the ring finger (3) relate to the lower section of the torso.

ods can reveal about the status of the body's qi. Just as a wine connoisseur can tell a wine's vintage, grape, and the manner in which it was fermented simply by tasting, a trained Chinese medicine practitioner can tell a lot about a person's qi through tongue and pulse diagnostic methods.

Acupuncture

In the introduction I briefly described acupuncture as a practice that restores the normal flow of qi through the channels (meridians) by stimulating acupuncture points. In the *Yellow Emperor's Classic,* this basic principle is carried to such complex levels that even longtime students of Chinese medicine find these materials difficult to fully understand. The essence of the information, however, is really quite simple: the qi of our external and internal environments continually evolves—rising, peaking, and declining. So long as qi is able to rise, peak, and decline without obstruction, it strikes a natural balance and allows us to achieve our full potential of physical, mental, and spiritual health. If our qi becomes obstructed—that is, it's unable to rise, peak, and decline freely—it causes an imbalance between yin and yang, which leads to an unnatural, unhealthy state.

The *Yellow Emperor's Classic* describes how to measure the evolution of qi when looking for signs of imbalance, and then how to employ methods such as acupuncture to help restore its normal flow. The qi circulatory system is described as being composed of 365 primary points along a complex network of twelve main and two special qi pathways. These acupuncture points are classified by how they affect the evolution (circulation) of qi throughout this network. If a person is diagnosed with too much second phase (mature yang) qi, for example, several acupuncture points known to help drain excess second phase qi can be stimulated. Because excess in one phase of qi usually indicates an accompanying deficiency in another phase, the best acupuncture points to treat this imbalance would be those that take from the excessive phase and give to the deficient phase.

Acupuncture points are therefore classified by how they affect rising, peaking, and declining qi that is continually evolving and circulating throughout the body. Some points help build a certain type of qi, while others may reduce it. Some points help shift qi from the primary channels to the organs, while others shift qi from the organs to the channels. Whether describing details of Chinese qi physiology, qi diagnosis, or acupuncture-point selection for treating qi imbalances, the complex details of the *Yellow Emperor's Classic* all follow the laws of Chinese science I have presented so far.

In a Nutshell

Acupuncture is a sophisticated branch of a profound science born in the mystical age of the ancient high civilizations. According to Chinese science, the material world around us is but the tip of the iceberg of what life is all about. In addition to the material realm, there coexists a realm of spirit and a mysterious force that bridges the two, which the Chinese call qi. Only in the last fifty years or so has Western science begun to discover many of the same notions of a continually evolving, holistically interconnected universe that Chinese science has long been based on. If Western science were ever to seriously address questions of spirituality, we might finally prove Mr. Kipling wrong and find the two sciences—East and West—meeting as one.

So how did the ancient Chinese develop a system of thought so advanced that in some ways it surpasses modern science? And how did they ever come up with the idea of sticking needles in people as a form of medical therapy?

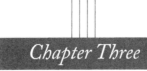

Chapter Three

THE SCIENCE

OF SORE SPOTS

Do a little reading on the subject of acupuncture and you are likely to run across a significant discrepancy. Some sources proclaim acupuncture to be five thousand years old while others say it began around three thousand years ago. A third date of just over two thousand years is just as likely to be cited. The five-thousand-year dating is based on traditional folk history, especially the legends regarding the Yellow Emperor. The more conservative three-thousand-year and most conservative two-thousand-year dates are the ones modern scholars use based on specific evidence.

There are disagreements among scholars over how to interpret some of the earliest known records that may refer to the practice of acupuncture. This discrepancy mostly revolves around the translation of passages in written historic records dated around 500–600 BCE.

One group of scholars cites these passages as mentioning acupuncture, while others translate these passages differently and do not think acupuncture is being discussed. The more conservative scholars say that the earliest definitive reference to the practice of acupuncture in available literature (which includes the compilation of the *Yellow Emperor's Classic*) dates to the second century BCE.

Complicating the question of when acupuncture began is the fact that no one seems to know *how* it first began. My research over the years has turned up four theories that pertain to the origin of acupuncture. There is an old legend that tells a tale of an ancient soldier who was cured of an illness after being shot with an arrow. A scholar who specializes in the study of Chinese medicine recently speculated that acupuncture might have its roots in a type of ancient exorcism in which a shaman uses a lance or sword to scare away evil spirits. This same scholar and others also think acupuncture may have evolved from the practice of bloodletting. Finally, there is an obscure reference, credited to the great Taoist sage Lao Tzu, which says that the ancient Chinese noticed that when people became ill they developed sore spots that later vanished when their illness subsided.

The first theory—that of the ancient soldier and his lucky arrow—is the one found most often in nonscholarly sources. I have never run across any specific details associated with this theory such as what region of China this incident was supposed to have occurred in or what kind of problem was supposedly cured. Most legends of important people or events usually contain ample details to support the main theme—although these may vary as the legend is retold. The lack of details associated with this legend causes me to wonder if this theory might not have been a wild guess someone once made when trying to imagine how the idea of poking needles in people began. If no other credible theories were put forward to challenge this one, it may have survived over time by default.

The theory that the inspiration for acupuncture may be traced to rituals utilizing swords or lances to chase evil spirits away was suggested by the historian Paul U. Unschuld in his book *Medicine in China a History of Ideas* (Berkeley: University of California Press, 1985). Unschuld is a strong proponent of the more conservative translation of ancient passages and disagrees with those scholars who trace acupuncture back to nearly three thousand years ago. While Unschuld offers his theory as a possibility, he is not insistent on the idea and says flatly: "The origin of acupuncture in China is not clear" (p. 94). Unschuld also thinks the theory that acupuncture evolved from bloodletting is a viable possibility.

While not wishing to discount these three theories entirely, I believe the theory attributed to Lao Tzu dealing with sore spots is the most plausible. The mystic sage Lao Tzu, who lived around 500 BCE, is credited with being the father of Taoism and writing the well-known book the *Tao Teh Ching* (pronounced *"dao duh ting"*)—the source of the saying "A journey of a thousand miles begins with a single step." Few people, however, are aware that there is another book attributed to Lao Tzu known as the *Hua Hu Ching*, which translates as *The Classic of Refining and Transforming the Rough and Undeveloped*. I began my study of this book in 1978 when I took a series of classes on it from Master Ni as he was readying his translation of this work for publication. He published this translation in 1979, together with his translation of the *Tao Teh Ching*, under the title *The Complete Works of Lao Tzu*. Master Ni's publication was the first English translation of the *Hua Hu Ching* and was perhaps the only complete copy of this teaching anywhere in the world.

The format of the *Hua Hu Ching* is that of a dialog between Lao Tzu and a bright student, very much like the dialog between the court physician and the Yellow Emperor in the *Yellow Emperor's Classic*. In the fourteenth century, Emperor Shuen Ti ordered the *Hua Hu Ching* destroyed, as some believed the student being taught by Lao Tzu might have been the Buddha (although this is not written in this book). As Buddhism was the prominent religion in China at that time, religious leaders felt such beliefs would undermine the authority of Buddhism and convinced the emperor to destroy this ancient text. It was only through oral transmission within Master Ni's Taoist lineage that he was able to translate and publish this work.

The *Hua Hu Ching* is a comprehensive treatise on profound spiritual concepts that form the core of Taoist philosophy. In one section of this work, Lao Tzu briefly describes twenty "Taoist holistic sciences," including "yi yau," the science of healing. Here Lao Tzu was recorded as saying:

> The ancient sages intuitively discovered that there were certain points on the body which became tender when the person became ill. When the illness had gone away, the tenderness was also gone. They discovered that by manipulating these points they could influence the internal organs and thus cure the disease. This is how acupuncture and acupressure developed. (*The Complete Works of Lao Tzu*, translated by Hua-Ching Ni, 1st ed. [Los Angeles: *Shrine of the Eternal Breath of Tao*, 1979], p. 142.)

The main reason I consider the theory regarding sore spots the most likely is the experience I have had learning and practicing acupuncture and acupressure. In my practice, I sometimes refer to the work I do as the "science of sore spots," because finding and manipulating such spots is so instrumental to the services I perform.

HANDS-ON LEARNING

I first became interested in the subject of sore spots as a nineteen-year-old with a bad back who happened upon a book on "shiatsu," a style of Japanese acupressure. Shiatsu is a method that employs rather forceful pressure, mostly with the thumbs, directly on established acupressure points. The author of this book recommended learning how to gauge the amount of pressure one would apply by practicing pressing one's thumbs on a bathroom scale. Some points may call for ten pounds of pressure, for example, others fifteen or twenty.

After reading this book, I learned that a shiatsu master was to teach a class at an acupressure school nearby. The teacher, Wataru Ohashi, had been trained in Japan and eventually moved to New York and established an acupressure school there. Ohashi, we in this class were to learn, had recently undergone a revelation of sorts in his method of practice. While he had been trained in the classic shiatsu style of regulated pressure on established points, he had recently changed his style to one in which he used a very gentle, probing technique. This style was such a departure from what he had been teaching at his school that he began telling his past graduates that he had "taught them wrong."

A key aspect to Ohashi's new style was for the practitioner to become acutely aware of his or her patient's slightest discomfort. Rather than using a predetermined force on specific points, Ohashi taught us to gently probe all over the body and try to sense what spots caused any discomfort. Once such spots were found, the force applied was to remain just under that which would cause the patient's muscles to tighten in resistance. By patiently keeping the force just under the threshold of resistance, the patient's muscles would eventually relax, and deep pressure could be applied without having to use forceful pressure.

Ohashi taught that while classic acupressure points, those hundreds of dots that pepper figures on acupressure/acupuncture charts, were the most common areas where qi (ki) tended to stagnate, *any* point of tenderness was a sign of qi stagnation. As important as it may be to learn the location and indications of classic points, it was just as important to learn how to find sore spots wherever they may appear.

As our class was an introductory course, Ohashi concentrated in teaching his techniques for finding sore spots rather than teaching us details of classic point locations and indications. After completing this course, I began to apply what I had learned in the massage/acupressure sessions I preformed on friends and family, and especially on myself.

When I enrolled in acupuncture school some years later, I began an intensive study of nearly four hundred classic acupuncture points. I was taught to find these spots by virtue of their position in relation to anatomical landmarks, and such details as the depth and angle with which acupuncture needles were to be inserted. Choosing what points to use in treatment was done by assessing a patient's rising, peaking, and declining qi with pulse and tongue diagnosis (see chapter 2), as well as checking specific spots called "alarm" points. Alarm points are given that name because unusual tenderness at these spots serves as an alarm suggesting the patient may have a specific internal problem. When the illness associated with alarm points improves, the tenderness of these spots will fade—just as Lao Tzu was recorded as stating.

When I began my practice, I combined what I had learned and treated my patients with both acupuncture and acupressure/massage techniques. I like to think my training served me well. From Ohashi I learned how to touch my patients, seeking out sore spots wherever they might be, and working the soreness out with my fingers. In acupuncture school I learned the complex theories of Chinese medicine; diagnosis of qi imbalances, the qi circulatory system, how specific points can adjust qi circulation and restore balance, and how to find and manipulate those spots with hair-thin needles.

After I had been in practice a few years, I met someone who would help me take my practice to another level. Master Si-Tu Ji had been apprenticed to an elderly monk of the Shaolin order at the age of four and trained in a system of qi-gong (also spelled chi-kong). Qi-gong is both a system of exercises to maintain and restore health and another means by which a healer can manipulate a patient's qi. As an exercise, qi-gong is similar to tai chi—a series of intricate movements designed to balance one's body, mind, and spirit by unblocking obstructions in one's qi circulation. After practicing such exercises successfully and improving one's qi circulation, some become very sensitive to other's qi blockages and can use this sensitivity in healing. Some qi-gong "masters" are thus able to use their qi to manipulate the qi of their patients.

After practicing several of Master Ji's qi-gong exercises for some two years, I experienced a sudden breakthrough in my own qi circulation system. I became very sensitive to my patients' qi blockages. While I had developed a pretty good ability to find classic points according to traditional locations and other sore spots by the gradual, probing style I learned from Ohashi, I suddenly found myself able to zero in on such spots within seconds. At first I was a bit hesitant to use my newfound sensitivity. I had spent years learning how to methodically diagnose my patient's qi imbalances and chose points by a combination of classic point prescription and whole body probing for hidden sore spots. Now I was finding points in seconds as though being drawn to them by some mysterious, magnetic force.

Master Ji helped me to feel more comfortable about utilizing my new sensitivity. He explained that this method of finding points was similar to finding where to dig a well by using divining rods—trusting one's intuition to pick up on very subtle signals. He had been taught that this method was how many of the acupuncture points were discovered in ancient times. Was this what Lao Tzu meant when he said the ancient sage "intuitively" discovered tender points that came and went with illness? As I slowly incorporated this new technique into my practice, I was pleased with the results and learned to trust my intuition regarding points.

Every day in my practice, the degree of help I was able to provide my patients hinged on my ability to draw upon what I had learned and successfully find and manipulate acupuncture/acupressure points. I came to believe the phenomena of sore spots appearing and disappearing with illness held the key to understanding how this practice may have begun. Exploring this hypothesis, I eventually developed a theory of a sequence of events leading up to the discovery of sore spots, as described by Lao Tzu, and perhaps eventually leading to the practice of acupuncture.

▪ DID IT ALL BEGIN WITH A BOO-BOO? ▪

If you have ever had a full body massage, chances are your massage therapist found several sore spots scattered throughout your body in places you never suspected were sore. I find such spots on my patients every day in my practice, often within seconds of running my hands over them. I call these "hidden" sore spots because a patient will not be aware of them until they are touched in just the right way. I will help you to locate some of these spots for yourself in chapter 9.

Hidden sore spots often feel like a deep bruise, even when pressed with very little pressure. Most who experience this during a massage assume that these spots are just minor strains within their muscle fibers, and sometimes that is all they are. Some of these spots however, are actually of the type described by Lao Tzu—unusually tender areas that mysteriously arise sympathetically with other problems.

How did the ancient Chinese first discover the relationship between these spots and illness? The answer may lie in a phenomenon all of us have experienced but few of us have seriously considered, namely: rubbing a boo-boo makes it feel better.

Bump your head or elbow, and you will automatically reach to rub it. The same thing goes for a sore muscle or joint—humans have an urge to touch and rub sore spots. This action is probably instinct, although my research has been unable to confirm this. Whether it is instinct or learned, somehow rubbing these spots makes them feel better. The next time you bump yourself in this way, try to avoid the urge to rub it. You will find it hard to resist, and when you don't rub the spot the pain will seem to last longer.

Virtually every traditional culture employs some form of touch therapy, and it is reasonable to assume these practices might have their roots in the urge to rub sore spots. Life in prehistoric times was difficult, and comforts were few. Depending on how far back one believes we can trace the human family tree, we can say with certainty that our earliest ancestors survived hundreds of thousands if not millions of years without clothing, the construction of dwellings, or the use of fire. Sore muscles and joints must have been common, and these early people would have found that rubbing these areas brought a welcome measure of relief.

Rubbing a sore spot (let's call this the "primary pain") helps it to feel better but may not take it away entirely. Continue to probe beyond the area of the primary pain, as I learned how to do from Ohashi, and you will find "hidden" sore spots. Hidden sore spots on the hip or elbow, for example, often accompany a primary pain in the shoulder. At first the relationship between hidden sore spots and primary pains undoubtedly went unnoticed. Eventually though, after observing such spots appearing and disappearing together with primary pains, someone came up with the idea that such spots might be related.

After the prospect that hidden sore spots might be related to primary pains dawned on our ancestors, the next step would have been experimenting with rubbing out the soreness of hidden sore spots to see if that would help the primary pain. It did! Rubbing out the soreness of the spots on the hip or elbow that arise with a shoulder pain does indeed help the shoulder pain feel better. The discovery of hidden sore spots' relation with primary pains and their therapeutic value may well have been one of the most significant discoveries of ancient time, as it spawned a healing system that has survived thousands of years and has helped countless millions.

While Lao Tzu described the discovery of hidden sore spots being related to illness, I feel it is more likely that this discovery first took place in conditions involving pain, as I just described. The association of sore spots and other types of illness would have been the next major milestone. Once the ancients learned the value of hidden sore spots in treating aches and pains, they probably would have spent more and more time looking for these spots and their association with primary pains. At some point, it must have been noticed that hidden sore spots spring up on individuals who did not have any pains but suffered other illness. Hidden sore spots on the chest, upper back, and wrists, for example, often accompany a cough. When the cough subsides, so too will the soreness of those spots. Rub out the soreness of those spots, and the cough will improve faster than expected, just as rubbing out the soreness of the spots associated with primary pains helps them to subside.

With this series of events, the ancients had discovered a valuable tool to aid their struggle for survival and improve the quality of their lives. I like to refer to primitive touch therapy as the "tool of touch" because I believe it was as valuable to our early ancestors as was the discovery of how to make stone tools. The more they learned about where hidden sore spots could be found, what conditions these spots were related to, and how to stimulate these spots with their fingers, the better they were able to treat a wider range of problems. Lower primates—chimpanzees and so forth—are known to spend hours grooming one another. The early pioneers of touch therapy, possessing larger brains and greater finger dexterity than other primates, probably spent a good deal of their free time massaging their sore muscles and joints, perhaps even doing this on each other in regular massage sessions as lower primates do in regular grooming sessions. This early stage would have been similar to the probing style of acupressure/massage I first learned before I was taught the locations of established points. Eventually, certain members of each tribe who excelled at the art of touch therapy probably emerged and were recognized as healers.

EARLY WARNINGS

As generations of tribal healers continued to refine their ability to find and manipulate sore spots, they made the next milestone discovery: hidden sore spots can appear before the onset of pain or illness. The alarm points I mentioned earlier not only are checked to help confirm the reasons for a current illness but also can sometimes serve as an early warning of an underlying qi imbalance that could signal a coming illness.

How could primitive people have discovered something so sophisticated? When performing regular maintenance touch therapy on healthy subjects, a healer may find hidden sore spots that do not seem to be related to any health problems. Finding new hidden sore spots on a subject who does not have any known pains or symptoms of illness is not unusual. As I mentioned earlier, sometimes these spots are just minor strains within muscle fibers. These spots heal quickly and are not related to other physical problems. Some ancient healers must have noticed however, that certain subjects with these "unrelated" hidden sore spots later developed a pain or illness that the hidden spots were related to. Hidden sore spots on the chest, upper back, and wrists, for example, are found on a member of the tribe who does not have a cough; then, some days later, this person develops a cough.

As with the earlier discoveries, once a connection was suspected between sore spots and health problems, the next step would have been manipulating those spots to try to relieve the problems they were related to. Finding hidden sore spots on the chest, upper back, and wrists, the healer rubs the soreness out of these spots. Over the next few days, most of the members of the tribe come down with a cough while the one who had the preventative therapy does not. Once a healer had seen this happen enough times, he or she would become convinced that rubbing such presymptomatic sore spots helps to prevent the onset of illness.

Over perhaps dozens or even hundreds of generations of refining their skill in touch therapy, the ancient Chinese had developed means to treat both pain and illness and even to predict and prevent some disorders. They had not yet, however, discovered acupuncture. In order to understand how the ancient Chinese may have made the leap from using their hands to using needles, I will need to explore in more detail the nature of sore spots.

GETTING TO THE POINT

Most people have had the experience of rubbing a sore muscle and finding a small spot that seemed to be the source of the larger area of pain. People often call this a "knot." Zeroing in on this spot directly provides more relief than rubbing the larger area of pain. What most people do not realize is that within that knot there will be a smaller spot. This smaller spot may be no bigger than the head of a match but will be surrounded by a protective layer of tight muscle, making it difficult to detect. Skilled touch therapists learn an array of techniques to relax muscle fibers surrounding these spots so that they may touch them more directly.

Touch therapy is much more effective if one can uncover the match-head-sized spots buried within knotted muscles. This is true both for primary pains and associated hidden sore spots. Being able to find and manipulate these spots takes a combination of a natural ability, training, and experience. In chapter 2, I used the example of a skilled wine connoisseur as someone able to detect things most of us could not. The same applies for someone skilled in touch therapy. It is possible to develop one's sense of touch to the point that one is able to feel things others cannot detect. Sightless people, for example, often develop a heightened sense of touch. In Japan, some of the most respected acupressurists are sightless. While finding sore spots no bigger than a match-head buried within a muscle takes a refined sense of touch, the match-head-sized spot is not the end of the story. Within the match-head spot, there will be an even smaller spot not much bigger than a grain of sand.

The vast majority of sore spots, however large an area of discomfort they cause, are the result of tiny problem spots literally the size of a grain of sand. These spots are the true epicenters of the soreness. Many people have rubbed their own aching muscles, but few have developed their sense of touch to the degree of being able to feel tiny problem spots the size of a grain of sand. I am not able to tell the vintage or age of a wine by tasting it, but I understand there are those who can. I am, however, able to find tiny sore spots on virtually anybody I work on, just as many other acupuncturists and acupressurists can. Of course most people, including most medical doctors, have not developed their ability to feel such fine spots. But just because relatively few people have this capability does not mean such spots don't exist.

Once the ancient Chinese healers had refined their sense of touch to such a fine level, they would have also learned how difficult it is to manipulate these tiny spots with their fingers. While it is possible for a touch therapist to use a portion of a fingertip to apply pressure directly to a match-head-sized spot, you cannot make your fingertip small enough to zero in on the grain-of-sand-sized epicenter. I discovered this for myself after some years of refining my skills in the probing style of acupressure/massage I learned from Ohashi. Feeling these tiny problem spots encased in muscle fibers, you find yourself wishing you had some sort of ultrathin device, an extension of your fingers that could glide through the overlying fibers and reach that spot—a needle! I believe a desire to reach such spots is how the acupuncture needle came to be used—as a tool touch therapists used to help them reach tiny, elusive problem spots.

Just as touch therapy is most effective when the therapist is able to zero in on problem spots with the fingertips, acupuncture is most effective when the acupuncturist is able to find grain-of-sand-sized spots with the tip of an acupuncture needle. Once a needle has been inserted through the skin and into the muscle, acupuncturists often employ a sort of "hunt-and-peck" technique. The needle tip is raised and lowered slightly several times, each time moving the needle tip ever so slightly from where it was before. When the tip of the needle is moved into just the right location, the patient will feel a sudden jolt—like two magnets, inched into their range of attraction, suddenly snapping together as one. Often, the acupuncturist will also feel a tiny jolt through the needle. This sudden reaction signals that the bull's-eye (grain of sand) has been found. It is quite remarkable how moving the tip of a needle just a hair can make such a big difference in the degree of sensation a patient feels. Touch the match-head spot with the needle tip, and the patient feels something—hit the grain of sand, and they feel a strange, painless jolt.

EARLY NEEDLES

Legend has it that early acupuncture needles were made of slivers of bamboo and carefully selected fish bones. Either of these two instruments would have made good needles in that they are thin, sharp, and flexible. Unfortunately, these perishable instruments could not survive the ravages of time, and even if they did and we were lucky enough to find any of these instruments, it would be impossible to prove they had been used as acupuncture needles. At times I have used the terms the "tool" of touch and the "art" of touch therapy to describe this subject. Unfortunately, unlike the study of stone tools or ancient works of art, we can never hope to find those first generations of acupuncture needles to help us trace the evolution of prehistoric touch therapy into the practice of acupuncture.

A central feature of our ancestors' gradual refinement of tool-making was the increasing sharpness of these instruments. By 20,000 years ago axes, knives, scrapers, and the like were being produced with edges that were literally razor sharp. Different types of perforators or needles also began to be produced, most likely for sewing animal skins. If these early human beings were practicing touch therapy during the same era that their increasing finger dexterity was allowing them to craft sharper and more pointed tools, it is very likely that healers became sharper and more pointed in their touch therapy. It is also reasonable to assume that if ancient touch therapists believed that the best spot to touch was too small for their fingers to reach, they would have looked to the tools they relied on in other areas of their lives and put the two together.

Records show that over time, needles made of flint (ouch!) and then eventually steel were developed, and that steel needles became favored as the most popular method to stimulate points. The *Yellow Emperor's Classic* makes no reference to acupressure. While there may have been several reasons for this, a primary one, I believe, was that acupuncture often gets the job done with less time and effort on the healer's part.

SORE SPOT DETAILS

Acupuncture/acupressure points are found within muscle (or tendon) fibers. These fibers are like the woven fibers of a rope; they derive their strength by distributing the load among many individual fibers working together as a team. The match-head- or grain-of-sand-sized spots I referred to feel like a small cluster of these fibers that, for whatever reasons, have coiled up—almost like a distraught person curling into a fetal position. This makes the muscle weaker and less flexible. It also causes pain—our body's warning that something is wrong. If you successfully manipulate these spots, they will start to uncoil, restoring the fibers to their normal more flattened positions and reducing or even eliminating the pain. This may happen at the time these spots are manipulated—like little chips of ice melting under the touch therapist's fingertips—or slowly over the next few days. Whether the process is immediate or delayed, skilled touch therapists develop a sense of whether their therapy is achieving the desired result of helping these fibers uncoil.

Acupuncture is remarkably effective in getting muscle/tendon fibers to uncoil, especially in hard-to-reach spots, but it also functions as a labor-saving tool. For example, an extremely effective touch therapy technique is to apply pressure to a sore spot and hold it there for several minutes. This often works better than continually kneading or rubbing such a spot. In the practice of acupuncture, once a needle is inserted and positioned so its tip lightly touches the grain-of-sand spot, it can be left in place for several minutes. This can be done to several spots at a time. During this time, the patient can be left to rest, freeing the acupuncturist to do something else such as treat another patient if desired. In touch therapy, however, the therapist must be physically touching the point and can only treat one patient and a limited number of points at a time.

When I was enrolled in acupuncture school, some of my teachers told me that it was old folk knowledge that acupuncturists tended to live longer than acupressurists. The theory behind this legend was that the less contact a healer had with patients, the less he or she would be affected by patients' imbalanced qi. If this is true, or at least was believed to be true, this may also account for acupuncture becoming more popular over time.

Today, due to acupuncture's effectiveness as a shortcut compared to touch therapy, many acupuncturists do not develop their hands-on techniques to a high level—just as a modern craftsman, trained to use power tools, may not learn how to use hand tools to the highest possible levels. Because of this, not all acupuncturists learn how to feel some of the subtle features that can be found within human flesh. Instead, schools like the one I attended teach acupuncturists how to locate classic points based on their relation to anatomical landmarks and then to carefully stimulate these points with needles until the desired reaction occurs. Conversely, because acupuncture carries risks involved with piercing the skin and requiring highly regulated training and licensing, most skilled touch therapists do not learn acupuncture. It is not really necessary for acupuncturists to learn higher-level touch therapy or touch therapists to learn acupuncture, but becoming proficient in touch therapy before learning acupuncture tends to make one inclined to believe that needles were a logical next step in the long evolution of touch therapy.

THE WHOLE AND ITS PARTS

In chapter 1, I mentioned the research being conducted by Zang-Hee Cho and others using advanced brain imaging. These researchers are finding that when acupuncture is applied at classic acupuncture points, it causes specific reactions in the brain that often relate to the traditional indications of that point—as with the point on the little toe stimulating the brain's visual cortex. This research strongly suggests there is merit to the age-old claim that stimulating one area of the body can regulate the functions of a different area of the body but leaves open the question of why this should be.

In chapter 2, I explained the basis for feeling the pulse or looking at the tongue as methods of diagnosis by introducing what I called the Chinese "holistic" theory. This theory holds that every part of the body is connected to every other part, as everything in Creation affects and is affected by everything else in creation. If it is true that every part of a whole system, such as an individual human being, is connected in some manner to every other part of that system, then the little toe *is* connected to the eyes. "But," you may ask, "why was it then that when Dr. Cho's research team stuck a needle in a toe not known to influence eye problems, it didn't stimulate the visual cortex? If every part of the body is connected to every other part, shouldn't every toe be connected to the eyes?"

The answer to this question is yes—every toe, indeed every cell of the body, is connected to the eyes. In fact, every cell of a body is connected to every other cell of that body. That is what the holistic theory is all about. The crucial aspect of such holistic interconnections, however, is that not all connections are equal. While the toe that did not stimulate the visual cortex was indeed connected to the eyes, the degree of that connection was not as strong as that of the little toe. To take advantage of the overwhelming consequences of holistic interconnectedness, one needs to weigh the practical degree, or the scale, of the connection.

In his book *Chaos: Making a New Science,* James Gleick describes how the cutting edge of modern science now accepts the concept of holistic interconnectedness, yet many scientists resent this idea. He recounts a professor, obviously frustrated by the "new" holistic worldview, telling his class that one does not have to account for the effects of every leaf falling from a tree on some small planet when trying to calculate the motion of billiard balls on a pool table on earth. "Very small influences," the professor tells his class, "can be neglected."

The professor is right—very small influences can be neglected, and that is why Cho's test subjects' visual cortexes neglected the influence of one toe but were stimulated by the influence of another. The ancient sages described by Lao Tzu discovered what points on the body had a strong enough connection with the internal organs to be useful as a form of therapy. They found these relatively stronger interconnections because these spots were found to become unusually tender during illness.

Human flesh, composed of skin, nerve, muscles and tendons, connective tissue, and so on, constitutes a "part" of the whole organism.

An important attribute of human flesh is its ability to feel sensations, including pain, which serves as a warning when something is wrong with that part of the body. If our flesh is injured or somehow compromised, we feel pain. When another part of the body is injured or compromised, that part may not signal us with pain. If our lungs become compromised, for example, they often signal us with a cough. If every part of the body is connected to every other part, then an abnormality anywhere, such as the lungs, will cause an abnormality everywhere, including the flesh. As flesh primarily signals abnormalities by developing pain, an abnormality in the lungs will cause sore spots in the flesh. However, because holistic interconnections are not equal throughout the whole, an abnormality in the lungs will only cause sore spots to develop in those specific areas of the flesh that have a relatively stronger connection with the lungs.

When the physics professor told his class that very small influences can be neglected in calculating the motion of billiard balls, he was essentially saying that the classic mechanical physics ushered in by Newton works perfectly well for solving many of our problems. He pointed out what many consider a weakness in the practical application of the holistic, interconnected model of nature—that if we believe everything both affects and is affected by everything else, we will be overwhelmed with trying to calculate the effect of every falling leaf. But what the holistic model really tells us is to keep an open mind when looking for interconnections. Useful connections may not only appear on the mechanical level of one part being directly connected to its neighbor. The ancient sages, blissfully ignorant of our modern notions of how the body "should" work, stumbled across these subtle but useful connections when they discovered hidden sore spots in some unlikely places. "A spot on the little toe connected to the eyes? Why not? If everything is connected to everything else, nothing should surprise us." That is why I said in chapter 2 that *the ability to learn the status of the whole from the study of any part is limited only by the individual's skill in deciphering the impressions the whole leaves on the parts.* The impressions are always there, some so small, it's true, they can be neglected. Knowing those impressions are there, however, should inspire us to leave no stone, or leaf, unturned in our search for useful interconnections.

▪ WHAT GOES AROUND, COMES AROUND ▪

The profound ramifications of the holistic model not only explain why hidden sore spots should manifest with pain or illness but also tell us why manipulating these spots can help improve such problems. Holistic interconnections, it seems, are a two-way street. If a problem in the eyes, for example, causes a hidden sore spot to develop on the little toe, then relieving the soreness of that spot on the toe will help relieve the problem in the eyes. The relief given to the hidden sore spot, however, must be through natural means. If you ingest a painkilling drug, for example, to artificially relieve the sore spot at the little toe, this will not help the eyes, as this type of relief did not come about through the body's natural interconnected healing processes. Sore spots can naturally be relieved through touch, and so this type of relief helps to reverse the problem that caused such spots to spring up in the first place.

To the best of my knowledge, no one has been able to definitively show in scientific terms why rubbing a boo-boo causes it to feel better. Perhaps one day, if we devote billions of dollars to researching this question, we may be able to understand scientifically why touch can heal pain. I suspect the answer to this is similar to what Cho's research is telling us about acupuncture's influence on higher brain centers. In the meantime, it seems common sense to assert that human flesh is very responsive to touch. Touch has a regulatory or normalizing affect on some of the aches and pains the flesh develops, and, owing to the two-way street of holistic interconnections, this explains why touching hidden sore spots—with one's fingers or the tip of a needle—can help a wide range of different problems.

Countless generations of touch therapists refined and passed down what they had learned about sore spots. Eventually, the most commonly found points came to be designated the classic or "primary" points now found on acupuncture/acupressure charts and models. Later generations of therapists would be taught how to find the most common points and the conditions they arose with. By the time of the *Yellow Emperor's Classic*, however, these points were not chiefly classified by the conditions they were related to. As I mentioned in chapter 1, the acupuncture points described in the *Yellow Emperor's Classic* were classified by how they affected rising, peaking, and declining qi throughout a vast qi circulatory system—leaving one to wonder how such complex, holistic theories evolved.

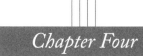
FIVE TO GO

During a class in 1977, while describing the important role the sun, moon, stars, and planets played in the lives of the ancient Chinese, Master Ni said something that planted a seed in my mind that continued to germinate for several years. He said that the idea for the concept of the five phases was inspired by the ancients' discovery of the orbits of the five planets, referring to the only planets that can be seen from earth with the naked eye. This tidbit of information struck me as remarkably important, although I did not know why. I also doubted historians would take this revelation seriously, as it was handed down as oral folk history with no written evidence to back it up. Ten years later, however, I ran across a passage in a book written by the great scholar, historian, and authority on ancient myths Joseph Campbell that also placed a great importance on the discovery of the orbits of the five planets in ancient time. Campbell credited this discovery as being pivotal to the sudden rise of the first high civilization in Mesopotamia some five thousand years ago. Just as important as the discovery itself, according to Campbell, was the notion held by the Mesopotamians that "the laws governing the movements of the seven heavenly spheres should in some mystical way be the same as those governing the life and thought of men on earth" (*The Masks of God: Primitive Mythology* [New York: Viking Press, 1959], p. 147).

The holistic science described in the *Yellow Emperor's Classic* was undoubtedly influenced by the same notions Campbell described— the idea that the natural laws that govern the movements of the heavenly spheres also govern the human organism. The quest to discover the order of the heavenly spheres had begun naturally enough long, long ago when a desire for warmth and light spurred our ancestors to begin following the patterns of the sun and moon. They came to recognize that the moon followed a repeating pattern and eventually discovered the pattern the sun follows as it moves back and forth when rising on the eastern horizon. Remarkably, they also discovered that the stars followed a repeating pattern as they circle overhead at night. The discovery of these repeating patterns had a tremendous impact on the thinking of our ancestors, as it fostered a sense of order within nature that *their* early ancestors had not enjoyed. Their fascination with following the movements of the heavenly spheres became intertwined with their spiritual beliefs, and they came to view the lights in the sky as reflections of the mind of God. Eventually, they developed abstract, numeric systems to help them follow and predict the patterns of the sun, moon, and stars—at least, most of the stars. Five stars did not follow the repeating pattern of all the others; they seemed to wander about the sky without rhyme or reason. These were the five planets (the word "planet" means "wanderer"), and figuring out their patterns was the last piece of a profound puzzle the ancients worked on for thousands of years.

During the same era, our ancestors learned to make an array of tools and developed methods to care for their sick. They even learned to manipulate their natural environment as a means of producing food by cultivating crops and breading animals. This led to a population explosion and created a host of new problems associated with large populations being tethered to relatively small areas of land. The need developed to organize human endeavor in ways never known before: in public works projects requiring unprecedented levels of cooperation, in accounting systems utilized in trade and taxation, and in formal systems of measuring time and space. There was also a need for leaders who could inspire the masses and earn their trust so as to steer them through these difficult times.

A new class of leader emerged during these tumultuous times that would prove both a blessing and a curse. Whether called "king," "pharaoh," or "emperor," such leaders were venerated as humankind's connection with the spiritual aspect of life. Virtually every ancient high civilization would have such leaders, and their power would be seen as absolute. How was it that these individuals came to be so venerated and elevated over everyone else to such a lofty position? Did they raise armies and force people to follow them? No. They were seen as the link between humankind and the spiritual realm because they held the key to solving the riddle of the five wandering stars.

Over countless generations, ancient astronomy, the study of the movements of the heavenly spheres, spawned ancient astrology, the concept that the position of these spheres, especially the five planets, influenced the destiny of human life on earth. Modern scientists tell us that the position of the planets cannot have any influence on human destiny. They point out that we now know that there are countless galaxies with billions of planets that ancient astrologers were unaware of, not to mention the three additional planets in our own tiny solar system the ancients could not see to take into account. They remind us that these ancient ideas were formed before we came to understand those spheres to be nothing but the residual elements of the Big Bang, drawn together by gravity.

Regardless of what we may think about the subject of astrology today, ancient people were convinced that heavenly supernatural forces held sway on earth and that humans could know something of the will of such forces by understanding the order of the heavenly spheres. The most mysterious and difficult to understand of those spheres were the five wanderers. The mysterious nature of these five convinced the ancients they represented the key to understanding the highest knowledge humans could possibly attain. When at last ancient astronomers finally solved this riddle, it was seen as cracking the code of God, and the ones who could decipher this code were the ones who could pass the will of God to the masses.

In China the emperor would be recognized as the one responsible for carrying out the "mandate of heaven." Before the term "emperor" was used, the original term for this top position was "di" (sometimes spelled "ti" but pronounced *dee* or *tee*). Historians tell us the original meaning of the term *di* has been lost over time, but this, like many insights regarding the crucial period prior to Chinese written history, has been handed down through Master Ni's oral tradition. The term *di* originally designated the stem of a fruit. The stem connects the fruit to the tree, allowing the essence from the great tree with its roots, trunk, and branches, to produce the fruit. The ancient Chinese saw human life as the fruit and the great spiritual realm as the tree. The fruit's stem, or "di," serves as the all-important middle ground (as discussed earlier) connecting the "yang" tree with the "yin" fruit.

The Yellow Emperor, or Huang Di, was the Chinese people's first formally recognized "di." As the one credited with inventing the compass and calendar, he was viewed as the one who best understood the movements of the heavenly spheres. Later generations of emperors would continue the tradition of managing the calendar, the instrument that became invaluable to populations dependent on plant cultivation. It is said that absolute power corrupts absolutely, and this unfortunately proved to be the case with later Chinese emperors, as it did with pharaohs and similar leaders in other ancient high civilizations. For the Chinese, these later generations of dis would begin to abuse their position and force the people to follow their rule under threat of violence. These leaders had lost the "Tao" and marked the end of China's golden age of virtuous leaders.

When Joseph Campbell traced the explosive growth of the first high civilization to the discovery of the orbits of the five planets and the related idea that human life should follow the order of the heavens, he was not just describing a time when ancient astronomers finally figured out these orbits. He was describing the crucial last component that led to humankind's greatest paradigm shift. As is the case with all paradigm shifts, no signal event can be credited with causing such great change. Many factors had been building for thousands of years, and the discovery of the orbits of the five planets brought those factors to a head. Before I go on to consider the ramifications of this paradigm shift, though, it is necessary to consider the additional technological innovations that allowed our ancestors to finally solve the riddle of the five wanderers.

REFINING THE YARDSTICK

Nothing about the appearance of the five planets readily distinguishes them from the thousands of stars scattered across the night's sky. Like those stars, the five visible planets—Mercury, Venus, Mars, Jupiter, and Saturn—appear as small twinkling lights of varying degrees of magnitude. The only thing different about these five is the fact that they do not hold their positions along with the other rotating, so-called fixed stars.

Once our ancestors made the remarkable discovery that the stars of the constellations rotated in a fixed pattern and then later realized there were five exceptions, they encountered significant obstacles trying to figure out the orbits of these five. Their orbits vary greatly, from as little as eighty-five days in the case of Mercury, to as long as nearly 29.5 years (10,750 days) for Saturn. Each of these five periodically undergo what is called "retrograde motion" where they appear to observers on earth to stop moving and then reverse direction before stopping again and resuming their forward motion. In order for our ancestors to learn their orbits, they needed to develop sophisticated and highly accurate methods for measuring the positions of the heavenly spheres.

One method our ancestors used to help orient themselves to the night sky was imagining the stars as groups or clusters that looked like different objects; a bear, a fish, and so on. Different tribes of peoples imagined different groupings, seeing different shapes in them. These groupings came to be known as constellations. The next step was conceiving the sky as being like a disc or sphere that rotated in a fixed pattern. The important aspect of this practice was the idea that observers could know the locations of all star groups at all times. Because their order was fixed—the first constellation always followed by the second, then third, and so on until the first comes around again—finding any constellation would let one know where all the others were.

While astronomers in different ancient high civilizations imaged different images and numbers of star groups, most eventually took the next giant leap forward by subdividing the spinning celestial sphere into 360 degrees. It is impossible to know whether this idea started in one culture and was spread to others or if different cultures came up with the same system of division independently. The concept of a circle or sphere being divided into 360 degrees is believed by experts to be a reflection of the other pivotal numbering system developed by certain ancient high civilizations in addition to the decimal system. This system, based on the number 60, is used to measure time and space and is known as the "sexigesimal" system. Even before the 60-based sexigesimal numbering system was formalized, I believe an important observation made by the ancients may have been the original inspiration for the concept of 360 degrees constituting a full circle.

One of the most important discoveries our ancestors made in their quest to follow the patterns of the heavenly spheres was that the sun moves back and forth with the seasons along the eastern horizon as it rises at dawn—eventually moving from one extreme point on the horizon to another and back. The two extreme points came to be known as the solstices, a phrase that means "sun stands still," as the sun would appear to stop moving at those spots for two to three days before reversing direction and resuming its movement. The full cycle of the sun's movement from one solstice point to the other and back takes 365 days and was recognized as constituting a complete cycle of the sun known as the "year." While observing this, our ancestors may well have counted the days by imagining each spot the sun first crested on the horizon as a specific point, or notch, on the horizon. Each "notch,"

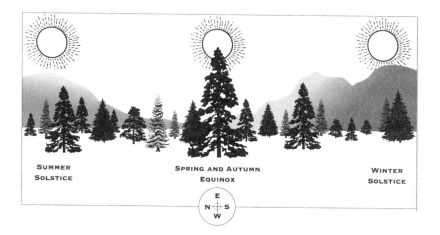

SUMMER
SOLSTICE

SPRING AND AUTUMN
EQUINOX

WINTER
SOLSTICE

E
N S
W

on the eastern horizon marked the location of that day's rising sun. Doing this, one would end up with very nearly if not exactly 180 notches, allowing for the fact that the sun would rise at the same notch during each solstice for two to three days. As the sun traveled from one solstice point to the other and back, it travels more than 360 notches.

Whether or not counting notches as the sun moved from solstice to solstice and back again was the original inspiration for conceiving 360 degrees as the circumference of a circle, this idea proved so valuable that we still use it today. By dividing the celestial sphere into 360 degrees, finer measurements could be made to aid the ancients' efforts to track the movements of the sun, moon, and planets relative to the "fixed" constellations. The 60-based numeric system would also prove quite popular and enduring. This system would later be used to designate the number of minutes in an hour and the number of seconds in a minute. The Chinese would base an important system for measuring yin/yang influences on this numeric system. They called this the "ten heavenly stems and twelve earthly branches"—often called the "stems and branches" system for short. The stems and branches figured prominently in Chinese astrology as the means to track the yin/yang influences of years, days, and hours. This system was also utilized in Chinese medicine, especially acupuncture.

THE YELLOW ROUTE

As the earth orbits the sun, it appears to earthly observers that it is the sun that constantly changes position. The ancients discovered that they could track this apparent movement of the sun in relation to the fixed constellations and that it repeated a pattern among those constellations every year. The yearly route of the sun among the constellations came to be known as the "ecliptic" in the West and was called the "yellow route" by the Chinese. Ancient astronomers found that tracing the ecliptic route allowed a more precise method for marking the solstices and equinoxes than did watching the back-and-forth movement of the rising sun on the eastern horizon. Eventually, measurements would be taken in which the ecliptic route served as a sort of baseline. It was found that the position of the planets always stayed fairly close to the ecliptic route, varying no more than about 8 degrees above or below it. This 16-degree band of sky became known as the zodiac in the West and was the area where ancient astronomers concentrated their observations, as this was where the moving heavenly spheres could always be found.

While Western astronomers divided the stars within the zodiac into twelve constellations and the Chinese divided them into twenty-eight constellations, both Western and Chinese astronomers came to divide the band of the zodiac into twelve sections, each one consisting of 30 degrees, making the complete 360-degree circle of sky that contained the moving celestial spheres. The Chinese divided the yellow route (ecliptic) into twenty-four seasonal periods of 15 degrees each; these twenty-four represented the yin/yang aspects of the more essential twelve divisions of 30 degrees. While the Western and Chinese astronomical systems had some differences between them beyond the number and makeup of their respective constellations, both shared the same basic numbering systems to orient observers to the heavens (see the illustration on page 58). With the aid of these systems, accurate measurements of the heavens could be made, including those of the five wandering stars.

With the aid of these important advancements in their measuring systems, the ancients finally solved the riddle of the five wandering stars. Like the sun and moon, these five did indeed follow repeating patterns. There were now *seven* moving heavenly spheres whose positions could be taken into account when trying to calculate the influ-

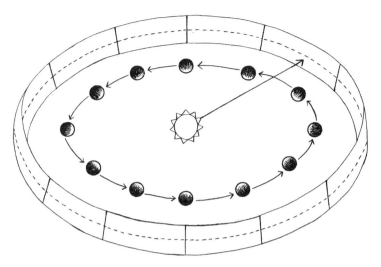

The apparent path of the sun was considered a central baseline from which observations of the stars and planets were made. This path came to be known as the ecliptic in the West and the yellow route by the Chinese. It was discovered that the movements of the five planets stayed close to the ecliptic, and an imaginary band above and below the ecliptic was envisioned and divided into the twelve sections known as the zodiac.

ence of the heavens. Being able to account for the positions of these seven and understand what those positions might mean to human life was the highest science of ancient time. Knowing their positions helped to refine the ability to predict weather patterns. It also spawned the belief that one could know something of their influence on human destiny. Whoever was in control of this knowledge had ultimate power.

CYCLES WITHIN CYCLES

It is difficult for us today to appreciate just how overwhelming the development of ancient astronomy was for our ancestors. The capability to trace the movements of these seven spheres pushed the human mind to develop its ability to think in abstract ways never known before. Developing the ability to count the number of days in the moon's cycle was a tremendous leap forward, as this gave our early ancestors their first yardstick with which to measure time. When the cycle of the sun was discovered, the complexity of the ancients' system for measuring time increased greatly, as the twenty-nine- to thirty-day cycle of the moon could now be contrasted with the 365-day (or so) cycle of the sun. One would not only be able to track events by virtue of their occurring on a specific day of the moon's cycle, such as a full moon but also one could now distinguish different full moons by virtue of what position the sun held that day. A full moon on the day of the summer solstice, for example, could be distinguished from a full moon when the sun was in a different position in its cycle.

The ability to contrast two different cycles greatly expanded our ancestors' ability to distinguish subtle differences between different days. This was crucial to the development of ancient astrology. As the orbits of each of the five planets were discovered and then confirmed one by one, these additional cycles could be contrasted also. When the orbits of all of the five planets were finally confirmed, this gave a grand total of seven cycles that could be contrasted against each other, creating mathematical possibilities that must have given ancient astronomers headaches.

Like any class of cutting-edge scientist, only a tiny number of our ancient ancestors had the ability to do the math needed to follow these cycles. Some ancient leaders had this ability themselves; others employed or otherwise held sway over those who did. The leaders who controlled this knowledge often proved it by ordering structures to be constructed that captured the positions of these spheres in predictable ways. All over the world, archeologists have found structures built in amazingly precise ways to capture specific rising or settings of the cycles of the sun, moon, and various planets. The appreciation of how important this practice was to ancient people has even led to the development of a new specialty in science known as archaeoastronomy, a combination of the fields of archaeology and astronomy. Scientists trained in astronomy and ancient astrology have proven invaluable in furthering our understanding of many archaeological sites and artifacts. While still in its infancy, archaeoastronomy promises to yield important new insights about our ancestors.

ON EARTH AS IN HEAVEN

The development of ancient astronomy pushed the envelope of early science. As often happens with scientific advancements, the new systems the ancients invented to help their quest to finally solve the riddle of the heavenly spheres ended up proving useful in many other important areas of life. All methods for measuring time and space can be traced back to this quest, as can the major systems of mathematics and accounting. The decimal and sexigesimal systems—indeed, the very concept of numbers themselves—all owe their existence to the same quest. How ironic it is that modern science finds astrology to have no credibility when there would be no science at all if not for the numbers, mathematics, and measuring systems our ancestor's belief in astrology spawned. With these innovations, all the features that constitute what is called "high" civilizations were made possible: large-scale public works projects, commercial trade and taxation, organizing large populations with common days of celebrations, and so on. All cultures that organize themselves with the aid of the compass and calendar, standardized weights and measures, numbers, and the mathematics they make possible owe this capability to the innovations of ancient astronomers who sought to solve the riddle of the moving celestial spheres.

Once this riddle was solved, ancient leaders organized society to mirror the order of the heavens. Archaeoastronomers can attest to the fact that many ancient civilizations went to great lengths to take the cardinal points of the compass and the light or shadows made during solstices and equinoxes into account when building pivotal structures or monuments. This was not only true for the pyramids or Stonehenge. Attention to such details can be found in the roads, burial sites, and temples of many cultures around the world, not to mention their arts. It is no exaggeration to say that for many of these cultures, astronomical/astrological concerns were the driving force behind their everyday lives.

In addition to spawning new technologies, knowledge and skills refined long ago would be molded to fit the now dominant model of heavenly order. Earlier people had learned how to build dwellings or ceremonial buildings, but now many were built in alignment with the compass and with doors or windows positioned to catch the light of solstices, equinoxes, or rising or setting stars. People had been making art for thousands of years, but now much of high civilized art would center on astrological themes. For the Chinese at least, earlier generations had discovered and refined their knowledge of manipulating sore spots. Now this knowledge would be organized under the same astrological themes that were being applied to all other aspects of life.

The practice of organizing existing knowledge under the new paradigm of following heavenly order explains why the *Yellow Emperor's Classic* describes Chinese medical concepts in the way it does: why yin and yang was thought to be the most essential system of categorization; why the five phases of energy evolution was seen as the primary system to decipher the dynamics of a constantly evolving natural order; why there are 365 acupuncture points on twelve primary and two special energy channels.

The holistic concept stressed within the *Yellow Emperor's Classic* of humans as a microcosm within the macrocosm of the universe is a direct reflection of the idea that society should follow the order of the heavens. This bold idea was considered absolute. Every bit of creation—from the smallest to the largest—followed this order, so human physiology must do the same. The job of the physician was first to learn the details of the dynamics of this absolute order, then practice recognizing how these factors were manifesting within their patients, and finally how to manipulate these dynamics to restore order.

The seven heavenly spheres held the key to understanding this universal order. People tend to get confused when trying to understand the different systems of medical thought described in the *Yellow Emperor's Classic,* in that some are based on even numbers traced to yin/yang categorizations and others use the odd-numbered five phases system. Recognizing that these systems can be traced back to the sun, moon, and five planets helps to clear up this confusion.

Understanding the relationship between yin/yang and the five phases in Chinese medicine is similar to understanding how the ancients viewed the seven spheres. The sun and moon were the first of these spheres to be recognized by the ancients and were seen as the most important of the seven. Similarly, the concept of yin/yang was the first recognized and by far most important in Chinese science. As I mentioned in chapters 1 and 2, the ancient Taoist concept of seeing all in nature as pairs of opposites was deduced from many factors— male/female genders, pairs of arms and legs, inhaling paired with exhaling, and so on. Out of all of these factors, the division of day and night, ruled by the sun and moon, figured most prominently.

The concept of the law of opposites became ingrained in the ancient's minds long before the cycles of the five wanderers were discovered. As the ancients were wrestling with what to make of these five, they were refining their methods to measure things by counting. They had noticed people had five fingers on each hand and five toes on each foot. The human body itself has four limbs connected to a fifth component, the central torso. People have five senses. Many plants have leaves displaying patterns of five. From these and other observations, it struck the ancients that nature tended to express itself in groupings of five. As the duality of yin/yang thinking was firmly entrenched as the overarching paradigm with which nature was viewed, the new idea of things being grouped in fives was seen as an extension of the basic yin/yang grouping, and the five wanderers were seen as an extension of the sun and moon.

In essence, the seven moving heavenly spheres really constituted two groups: the primary sun/moon pairing and the extended group of five. More specifically, as I said in chapter 2, a group of five was seen as consisting of two levels of yin and two levels of yang, with the fifth component being the neutral transitional phase. The system of the five phases of energy evolution was eventually formally developed as an extension of the yin/yang law of opposites paradigm, with its emphasis on categorizing the dynamic phases of nature's constant cycles of evolution. The sun and moon were thus the primary inspiration for the basic concept of yin and yang while, as Master Ni taught, the five planets inspired the idea of describing the constant rise, transformation, and decline of yin and yang as happening in five phases.

The 365 "primary" acupuncture points were identified as a direct reflection of the solar cycle of 365 days. Actually, some sources list the number of primary points at 360 or 361. I believe this discrepancy can be traced back to what I described earlier about counting the number of "notches" on the eastern horizon, leading to the concept of a circle being subdivided into 360 degrees. The number of days the sun is thought to "stand still" when rising at the solstices is difficult to fix. It appears to stay in that spot for two or perhaps even three days. This may have lead some to round off the "moving" days to 360 while others rounded off the still days at an even two, arriving at 361 moving days. Those small details aside, it can be said with certainty that the number of primary acupuncture points was fixed to reflect the days of the solar cycle, despite the fact that many more therapeutic points were known to exist. Those additional points were eventually classified as secondary or tertiary points so as to leave the first level of points in line with the solar cycle. All of these therapeutic points, discovered by

trial and error and originally classified according to the health conditions they were known to be associated with, were reorganized under
the new paradigm of following the heavenly order.

UNDERSTANDING PATHWAYS

In addition to the total number of primary points, the concept that
these points were pivotal spots along twelve primary and two special
qi pathways was also established to reflect astrological understanding.
When I first began trying to grasp the factors that led the ancient Chinese to organize the acupuncture/acupressure system as they did, I could
not see the logic of having the 365 points being divided among fourteen
qi pathways. It would have made sense if the 365 points were on twelve
pathways. One could then deduce that the pathways were linked to the
twelve lunar cycles (months) and this system was organized like a calendar reconciling the solar and lunar cycles. Having those points on twelve
primary and two special pathways did not make much sense to me.
What was the relationship between the solar cycle (365 points) and
twelve regular plus two special groupings? I found the answer to this riddle once again in teachings handed down in Master Ni's tradition.

The two special channels I refer to divide the torso exactly in
two—the all-important middle ground. One runs from the back side
of the rectum, up the center of the spine, up and over the center of the
skull, and then down to the roof of the mouth. This channel is called
the "du" channel in Chinese and the "governing vessel" in English. The
other channel begins from just in front of the rectum and runs up
the center line of the front of the torso, then up the throat, ending on
the tongue. This is called the "ren" channel in Chinese or the "conception vessel" in English. When the mouth and rectum are closed, these
two channels constitute one complete circuit connecting the left/right
and front/back halves of the body. These two channels are thought to

circulate the very core of the body's qi (see the illustration). The twelve regular channels connect to and spring off of the circuit made by these two special channels.

In the introduction to his translation of the famous ancient oracle the *I-Ching*, Master Ni reveals that the du and ren channels were originally conceived of as mirroring the "yellow route," or the ecliptic path of the sun. Earlier in this chapter, I explained that the ancient astronomers divided the ecliptic into twelve sections of 30 degrees each to help them monitor the planets. This system of organizing the movement of the heavens must have been what inspired the Chinese to organize their system of qi circulation within the body. This explains

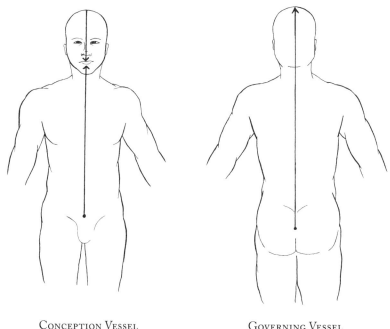

CONCEPTION VESSEL   GOVERNING VESSEL

The ren, or conception vessel, together with the du, or governing vessel, constitute a circuit that runs along the midline, dividing the torso and head in two. The other twelve primary qi pathways connect with this circuit. Note that the conception vessel drawing also shows the last section of the governing vessel.

THE HEALING POWER OF ACUPRESSURE AND ACUPUNCTURE

why there are twelve regular and two special channels. The twelve regular channels relate to the twelve divisions of the zodiac and the two special channels relate to the ecliptic.

The stars, once thought to be random, scattered lights, with no pattern, eventually came to be seen as important energy clusters (constellations) that were best understood by virtue of their relationship to the ecliptic route and its twelve subdivisions. The therapeutic points were likewise once thought to be random, scattered phenomena. Now, following the model used to solve the riddle of the heavens, they came to be seen as key energy spots within a holistically interconnected web that was also best understood as groupings around a central baseline made up of twelve subdivisions. Staying close to this baseline (du and ren channels) were the five special wanderers, represented by the five main organs within the torso (liver, heart, spleen/pancreas, lungs, kidneys).

Considering the foregoing, it becomes clear that when the *Yellow Emperor's Classic* refers to a human as a miniature model of the heavens, this was not just meant to be a vague, generalized analogy. The sun, moon, stars, and planets were believed to have quite real and specific correlations within the human body. The orbits of those spheres were thought to be manifestations of the circulation of qi within the heavenly body, and it was assumed the same pattern of qi circulation must also take place within the human body. Many acupuncture/acupressure points were seen as being to the human body what stars were to the body of the heavens. This can be seen in the fact that the term "celestial" ("tian" in Chinese) is the most common term used in the name of the primary acupuncture/acupressure points. In chapter 3 I explained that many of these points feel like tiny grains of sand within the muscles. They actually feel to one's touch the way twinkling stars look to one's eyes—like tiny kernels of energy. Modern scientists and songwriters alike tell us we are made of stardust. The ancient Chinese

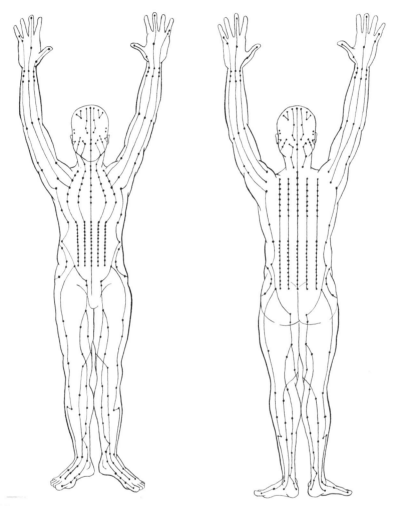

The ancient Chinese, following the model of the newly conceived system to organize the planets and constellations around the central line of the yellow route (ecliptic), organized the therapeutic sore spots into twelve regular pathways (meridians) surrounding the central line (ren and du meridians) dividing the torso.

believed humans were made of star qi, and their medical system became built upon this notion.

PUTTING IT ALL TOGETHER

Once the paradigm of heavenly order manifesting within the human body was established and the old therapeutic sore spots were looked at in a new light, theories about qi pathways were developed that helped to explain why these points had the functions they were known by experience to have. Why would stimulating a point on the little toe help the eyes as Cho's f MRI experiment sought to study? Because the point on the little toe is located on a qi pathway (subdivision) that connects that toe with the eyes via the brain. Future additions to Chinese medical theories would follow these astrological themes, whether they were organized under even-numbered yin/yang systems or odd-numbered systems based on five phases or the triad of yin, yang, and the harmonizing/transitional force.

Ironically, by the time the *Yellow Emperor's Classic* was written down and established as a definitive medical text just over two thousand years ago, the original astronomical and astrological inspiration for these concepts had long been forgotten. The core concepts—yin/yang, the five phases, and their related numeric systems—had survived the ages, but how these concepts first came to be was lost. This loss was very much like what happened in Egypt regarding the pyramids or in England regarding Stonehenge, where later generations were unaware of just how and why those structures were built.

So now, at last, we can see the logic behind the confusing theories of Chinese medicine. These ideas were not just pulled out of a hat by someone at some point in the past. They were based on the very same notions our ancestors developed to understand their complex natural environment and put the confusing world around them into a context they could grasp and pass on to others. Modern critics sometimes refer to Chinese medicine as based on superstitious notions. To that I would ask: "Is the calendar based on superstitions? Is the compass? Is our belief that there are four seasons superstitious or the notion that we can use numbers to understand nature?" As I will discuss in more detail in the next chapter, all of these concepts were tools that were developed following astronomical observations and astrological themes that helped our settled ancestors cope with modern (settled) life. They proved so valuable we still rely on them today without giving any thought to how they were developed and whether or not they reflect objective discoveries or subjective ideas that may constitute a type of superstition. These concepts proved equally valuable to the Chinese in their attempts to understand the complexities of human health and, like the compass and calendar, have continued to prove their value in each generation since their invention.

It may be impossible for us today to appreciate the connection our ancient ancestors felt with the heavens. For hundreds of generations, the lights in the sky were as important to them as the air they breathed or the food they ate. The ancients believed there was a power to those lights and the source of that power was the Creator of all within the heavens *and* on earth. As our ancestor's cognitive capacity grew and they began to recognize patterns to the movements of the heavens, their connection with the heavenly lights became more conscious. During the dawn of modern civilization, a unique balance was struck between the instinctual awe earlier generations felt toward those lights and the newer conscious understanding of their movements as being like a vexing riddle now solved.

During recent generations, modern science has seemed to take the awe and spiritual connection out of our appreciation of those heavenly lights. We have labeled such ideas as backward as our mechanical model of nature has sought to explain those lights as nothing more than nuclear reactions of elementary particles completely independent of the struggles of hominoids on one tiny planet among billions of galaxies. Ironically, as modern science presses on, there seems to be an interesting turnaround happening. The awe is returning to the science of the heavens. A new understanding of the enormity, complexity, and interconnectedness of the universe is occurring at the same time that the Hubbell telescope and other sources are capturing stunning images throughout the far reaches of space. Scientists are now able to witness the three stages of the birth, maturation, and death of stars and even whole galaxies. The majesty and magnitude of what is now coming to light is inspiring some scientists to see a divine hand behind the beauty of it all. If this trend should continue, future generations may once again be open to the idea of science and spirituality being combined, and medical models that seek to find a relationship between the order of the heavens and that of the human organism may not seem far-fetched at all.

Chapter Five

YIN/YANG THINKING

LEGEND HAS IT THAT WHEN THE Yellow Emperor was just sixteen years old, his tribe, the Han, was attacked by the combined forces of nine neighboring tribes. Even at this young age, the lad who would become the Yellow Emperor was respected as being very bright, physically capable, and sincere, and the members of his tribe asked him to lead the fight against their aggressors. After first suffering defeat, the Yellow Emperor prayed to the spirits of the Big Dipper and inspired his troops to do the same, and then his forces beat back the invaders. This legend underscores how deeply the ancient Chinese believed the lights in the sky were relevant to life on earth. His connection with the heavens was instrumental in helping his troops find the means by which to defeat their foes. The Yellow Emperor's understanding of the heavens also made him a quick study of healing knowledge, as this too was thought to be a reflection of celestial influences.

After uniting his people in this momentous defensive effort, the Yellow Emperor began to organize society with formal systems based on the order of the heavens. To do this, he sought the help of the best and brightest, especially the elusive sages—the Taoists—who chose to live as hermits in the high mountains, away from the growing settlements. In chapter 1, I explained the Taoist belief that humans once possessed a balance between their physical and spiritual (yin and yang) natures that was lost when the physical aspect of life was overemphasized. This loss of balance had begun by the time of the Yellow Emperor. The Taoist sages were those who had managed to maintain or restore their balance, and the Yellow Emperor sought their help so that he might bring a similar balanced approach to his administration.

Because of the Yellow Emperor's sincerity in seeking to help his people at this crucial period, the usually secretive Taoist masters were persuaded to share some of their ancient knowledge, including their insights regarding the order of the heavenly spheres. The hallmark of the Yellow Emperor's administration was his ability to pull together the profound knowledge of the ancients and incorporate this into social systems of a budding high civilization. The *Yellow Emperor's Classic* gives clues to his administrative style. The way he poses questions to his top court physicians shows that while he is sometimes quite knowledgeable about a given subject, he defers to the true experts. By asking pointed questions, he leads the expert to give details on subjects the Yellow Emperor has a general understanding of but of which he wants the details clearly laid out for the record.

As a result of his collaboration with the Taoist sages, the astronomically inspired concepts of yin/yang, qi, and the five phases were formalized, becoming the foundation of the Yellow Emperor's administration and the social customs of the Han people. Future generations would follow these customs until later leaders lost the Tao and the "golden age of sage leaders" succumbed to the inevitable decline (yin) that must follow all rising (yang). The decline that followed the loss of the golden age of sage leaders roughly coincided with the decline of the other ancient high civilizations such as the Egyptians or Minoans. Later generations of Chinese leaders held their positions by force instead of by virtue and claimed the mandate of heaven as the birthright of their kinship to previous leaders or through violent overthrow. With only minimal knowledge of the natural order, they followed superstitious beliefs in which demons and ancestral spirits ruled the world. However, because of oral knowledge passed down by Taoist sages through secretive sects, the principals of the Chinese golden age would resurface around 500 BCE, when the "Ageless Master," the venerable sage Lao Tzu, broke the secretive hermetic tradition and began to teach the ancient understanding openly to the people. In the centuries that followed, many of the ancient skills reemerged, although they never again truly became the norm for the masses nor the model for future leaders.

I believe it was during this stage that many ancient practices, including acupuncture and the theories behind Chinese medicine, once again began to find their way back to the people. The gap in the record that took place during the stage when such practices were limited to secretive traditions has caused later scholars to believe acupuncture was invented at this point of reemergence a little more than two thousand years ago. Modern scholars tell us the *Yellow Emperor's Classic* was compiled by various authors around 200 BCE and that these authors falsely attributed their ideas to the Yellow Emperor and his court to add more weight to their authority. Interestingly though, none of those who believe the practice of acupuncture and the theories behind it first sprang up at this time are able to shed any light on such fundamental details as how the acupuncture points were fleshed out, who those first authors may have been, or why they would have chosen to use a fictional leader from three thousand years in the past as the spokesman for a "new" system of healing.

YIN/YANG REVISITED

Regardless of differences of opinion over exactly when acupuncture was first used, who invented it, or what the original inspiration was behind it, it is clear that since the time of the *Yellow Emperor's Classic* the theories behind acupuncture revolved around the concept of yin/yang. I have discussed the yin/yang concept extensively but have not yet fully addressed its most profound (and slippery) aspect, namely, *what it tells us about how humans perceive the world around them.* A vital aspect of Taoist philosophy is contemplating the function of the mind. In earlier chapters, I explained the idea of a three-in-one and the pivotal role the balancing middle ground plays in this triad. Taoist philosophy teaches that while qi is the middle ground between the spiritual and material realms as a whole, the human mind represents the middle ground between a human being's physical body and spiritual nature. As the fulcrum between yin and yang, having a balanced mind is instrumental to reaching one's full potential. Because of this belief, an important but easily overlooked component of Taoist folk history involves tracing the evolution of human thought.

One of the foundations of modern science is the value it places on objectivity. Scientists strive to remain as objective as possible, making their observations without preconceived notions. As highly as pure objectivity is prized however, it is virtually impossible to escape the influence of one's pervading cultural prejudices. We seem destined to have our vision stained by the subjective cultural dogma of whatever society and bit of time we happen to be born into as such factors permeate the basic perspectives with which we view the world around us. We are taught these belief systems as tiny children, along with our survival skills, before we have any chance to weigh such beliefs for ourselves in a mature fashion. Even Einstein was unable to see through old dogma when he failed to explore the possibility that the "fixed stars" are not fixed and that the universe is expanding.

Taoist folk history teaches that our early modern human ancestors were highly intelligent yet extremely innocent beings. For countless generations, they learned survival skills from their elders, but no one told them how to think of the world around them in any judgmental way because no one had yet formed such judgments. Taoists came to revere their prehistoric ancestors because they thought of them as humankind's only truly objective generations—free from the cultural prejudices that would dominate later times. Master Ni refers to these early beings as the only "true scientists"—meaning the only completely objective observers of nature. Over time these innocent beings did reach some conclusions about nature and humankind's place within the big scheme of things. They were the only era of humans to do this on their own—without being told how to apply their conscious judgment before they had matured enough to reach their own conclusions. The conclusions these true scientists reached would form the basis of what later generations would label "Taoism."

> Tao, as the absolute Truth of the universe, is elusive and evasive.
> Though it is elusive and evasive, it unveils itself as images and forms.
> Evasive and elusive, it discloses itself as indefinable substance.
> Shadowy and indistinct, it reveals itself as impalpable subtle essence.
> This essence is so subtle and yet is so real.
> It is the primary origin of the whole of creation.
> It existed prior to the earliest time and only its name is new.
>
> Excerpt from chapter 21 of the *Tao Teh Ching*, translated by Hua-Ching Ni

Lao Tzu is often identified as the founder of Taoism. While he may have been the first to use the term "Tao" in its current context, he traced his lineage back to the sages long before the Yellow Emperor. This lineage extends back into the age of the innocent-minded objective observers of nature who became aware of the evasive and elusive impalpable subtle essence that constitutes the primary origin of the whole of creation and would only later be identified as "Tao."

Before Heaven-and-Earth are born,
  there is something formless and complete in itself.
Impalpable and everlasting, silent and undisturbed, standing alone and unchanging,
  it exercises itself absolutely and generates itself inexhaustibly in all dimensions.
It may be regarded as the Mother of all things.
Far beyond mankind's relative mental comprehension,
  it can be referred to by no specific name.
Yet it may be identified as Tao,
  the absolute nature of the universe.

Excerpt from chapter 25 of the *Tao Teh Ching,* translated by Hua-Ching Ni

The sages concluded that the manner in which the Tao "exercises itself," generating everything around us, can be traced to the interaction between polar forces they ended up calling "yin" and "yang." This conclusion was heavily influenced by the factors I have already discussed: the sun and moon, the two genders among species, and so on. The process of generation was also called the "mystical intercourse" of yin and yang.

The subtle essence of the universe is eternal.
It is like an unfailing fountain of life
  which flows forever in a vast and profound valley.

It is called the Primal Female, the Mysterious Origin.
The operation of the opening and closing
  of the subtle Gate of the Origin
  performs the Mystical Intercourse of the universe.
The Mystical Intercourse brings forth all things from the unseen sphere
  into the realm of the manifest.
The Mystical Intercourse of yin and yang is the root of universal life.
Its creativity and effectiveness are boundless.

Chapter 6 of the *Tao Teh Ching,* translated by Hua-Ching Ni

While the sages' objective observation of the constant ebb and flow
of nature—the rising and setting sun, the waxing and waning moon,
the shifting tides, the changing seasons, and so on, inspired their
thoughts regarding the Tao and the polar forces of yin and yang, later
generation's awareness of the Tao declined as emphasis began to be
placed on physical/material developments. During this era, the rise of
subjective concepts and subsequent loss of objectivity occurred. According to Taoist folk history, the rise of subjective concepts, more
than any other factor, marked the decline of the golden era of innocence. In order to better understand this accounting of history, it is
necessary to clarify the difference between an objective observation
and a subjective concept. To do this, I will return to those all-important
methods our ancestors developed to measure time and space.

OBJECTIVE VS. SUBJECTIVE

In the last chapter, I mentioned how the observation that the sun rises
in a different location on the eastern horizon influenced the development of the calendar. The ancients' discovery that the rising sun keeps
shifting back and forth from one extreme point on the horizon to another is an example of an objective observation. Anyone observing this

would come to the same conclusion. The decision to single out a complete back-and-forth motion and consider it a "cycle" and designate this cycle as a unit of time (one year) was not an objective observation that all observers would necessarily agree on. Rather, the idea to label this as such was a subjective concept that was the product of human imagination rather than an objective feature of nature. Our ancestors did not *discover* that the solar cycle takes "one year" or that sunrise occurs on the "eastern" horizon. They invented formal, subjective concepts of time and space as a means to place the natural phenomena they observed into a framework they could comprehend and communicate to others.

Another example: there are not really four seasons in any objective sense; someone just made that up. We could just as easily say that there are two seasons or twenty-two. The same thing goes for compass directions. The idea that there are four cardinal directions in space is a subjective invention of human imagination. As with the seasons, there is nothing inherent in nature that demands we designate four directions in space. The fact that our ancestors chose to do so reflects a type of subjective thinking—a "formula of thought," if you will, that coalesced during the stage when the slowly brewing pressures of settled life, and even the more slowly brewing discoveries of celestial observations, reached a critical mass.

Some might think that concepts of time and space and the methods we use to measure these are a natural, objective function of the modern human mind—that we are "hardwired" to perceive the world around us in this manner. However, Taoist folk legends tell us this is not the case, and this is supported by evidence that suggests these concepts first appeared just before the rise of high civilizations a little more than 5,000 years ago, and certainly not before the end of the last Ice Age 10,000 years ago. When you consider that modern humans, *Homo sapiens sapiens*, emerged at least 150,000 years ago and had replaced all other forms of *Homo sapiens* by at least 30,000 years ago, it makes no sense to attribute the rise of these concepts to a natural function of the modern human mind. Rather, these concepts reflected this new subjective formula of thought I referred to and proved so useful they were formalized at this crucial period and then passed on to successive generations—up to and including our own.

One way to think of the impact this formula of thought had on human development is to compare the human mind to a computer. While computers have certain basic capabilities such as processing speed and memory capacity, they require programming to put these capabilities to use. The measuring concepts I refer to provided a powerful new programming for the human mind, allowing those who learned these systems to process data, so to speak, in a new and exciting way. The great practical value of this programming, together with the ease with which it could be passed on to others, caused it to spread like wildfire. Today, the vast majority of the world's people continue to utilize this system of thought without being aware that it is a subjective program.

The essence of this program is a very basic concept in which a pair of opposites are established and then measurements are made by contrasting these, that is, by virtue of where something sits in relation to those opposites. The manner in which the rising sun shifts back and forth on the eastern horizon is an example of this. The pair of opposites that is established is that of the two solstices—the northern and southern extremes of the sun's movement along the horizon. Individual days are then measured by contrasting these two; figuring where the sun crests on the horizon in relation to those opposites. The equinoxes, for example, are right in the middle of these two opposites. All ancient high civilization utilized this program. The compass points were established following the same formula: A pair of opposites consisting of north (inspired by the North Star) and south are established, and then an object's location can be established by discerning where it stands in relation to these two opposites. In the case of the compass, a second set of opposites was established (west/east), and the two sets were contrasted against each other. The process of subdividing one pair of opposites into two pairs of opposites is called quartering. Quartering, like slicing a whole pie into four sections, was the most common application of this programming, as can be seen not only with quartering space into four directions but also in quartering a year into four seasons. For the Chinese, quartering is also expressed in the concept of the five phases, as I mentioned in chapter 2.

THE FOREST VS. THE TREES

What this programming allows people to do is to break down the holistically interconnected world around them into more manageable bits—bits of measurable time and space. This seems natural to us today, but the practice of doing this marked a radical shift in human thought. As difficult as it may be for us to imagine, our precivilized ancestors did not have the mental programming that would allow them to perceive their environment as being made up of "individual" things. As an example of what I mean, consider the way we look at the "parts" that make up an individual human being. When we look at one of our fellow beings, we can identify many parts, such as 10 fingers and toes, 2 arms and legs, a torso, and so on. While we may label such things individual "parts," we understand that these parts are not really individual or separate. You would never see any of those parts, such as a few fingers or a leg, for example, walking around on their own. These so-called parts only exist as integral components of a whole, larger system.

Our precivilized ancestors looked at the world around them in the same way we look at the parts that make up a whole being. When they looked at a forest, for example, they could distinguish this tree from that tree and a deer over here from a bear over there, but they did not see such things as lone, individual phenomena any more than we would think of toes or a torso as individual. They saw all parts of the forest, including other people and the one doing the observing (oneself), as integral components of the whole forest. While such holistic concepts are becoming popular today, and people like to say things like "We are all part of the whole," statements like these are more a reflection of a hopeful attitude than the way we actually perceive ourselves in relation to our environment. When most of us look at a forest today we see deer, bears, and people as complete individual things that happen to be within the forest. We do not see them as being like the toes, arms, and legs of a whole being, as the ancients did. If we did, modern scientists would know there could be no such thing as an uninvolved observer of experiments. Our innocent-minded ancestors did not just talk the talk of holism—holistic interconnectedness was all they knew.

A human being is part of the whole, called by us the Universe, a part limited in time and space. He experiences himself, his thoughts and feelings, as something separated from the rest—a kind of optical illusion in his consciousness. (Albert Einstein)

When Einstein commented that the way we experience ourselves as individuals is a kind of optical illusion in our consciousness, he used terminology similar to that found in many Eastern traditions. Buddhists, for example, speak of the human ego as an illusion that blinds and thus separates us from the great whole. The idea that we as people are "individuals," separate from all others, is often referred to as an illusion or a dream in such cultures. We find similar themes among the few remaining hunter-gatherer tribes and other more simple settled cultures who see strong connections between individuals and their surroundings. Many of these cultures think of the earth as their mother, the sky as their father, and the animals and other living creatures as their bothers and sisters. The great Taoist philosopher Chuang Tzu, who expanded Lao Tzu's teachings and is considered the second most important figure in Taoist thought, taught this also. Chuang Tzu had a wicked sense of humor and was quite fond of teasing people about their certainty regarding their sense of individuality. In one teaching he challenges the notion that we are individuals by examining the question "Is Self so?" His most famous teaching is one in which he told of a dream he had after falling asleep in a field of flowers on a spring afternoon. He dreamed he was a beautiful butterfly floating upon breezes without a care in the world. When he awoke, he was not sure if he was a man awaking from a dream in which he was a butterfly, or if he was a butterfly dreaming he was a man.

ANCIENT ARTIST

Evidence of the shift in thought from people assuming the interconnectedness of all things to the "optical illusion" of seeing things as individual phenomena, separate from the observer, can be seen in the changes that took place in early artwork. We have only recently begun to appreciate the vital role art played in our most ancient ancestors' lives and how this may help us understand more about their thinking. A good example of the important role art played in expressing our prehistoric ancestors' thoughts can be seen in the rock engravings and paintings (known as petroglyphs to scientists and called yan hua in China) found on a mountainside in a region of Inner Mongolia known as the Yin Mountains. Many thousands of these carvings were made on a vast mountain face covering an area some 70 meters high and 120 meters wide. Even more remarkable than the sheer size of this site is the fact that these carvings were made over a period of some ten thousand years. Can you imagine any group of people doing anything continuously for ten thousand years? Millions of similar engravings and paintings have been found around the world.

While not as great in size, the most famous and impressive example of the highly sophisticated level of prehistoric art can be seen in the numerous cave paintings found in Europe, especially in France. Most of these paintings are buried deep within the bowels of interlocking caverns and required the artists or anyone who wanted to view these works to crawl hundreds of yards along narrow passageways to reach the pitch-black galleries. Art experts agree that these paintings, ranging in age from ten thousand to more than thirty thousand years, show true mastery of the concepts of form, space, and color. Some of these drawings even take advantage of contours of the cave walls, giving an almost three-dimensional effect.

One thing these cave paintings or rock art do not show, however, is any concept of a border within which to frame these works. Nor is there any sign of the concept of geometric shapes. In other words, there is no suggestion of the concept of circumscribing or dividing space—no attempt to carve out a measured bit of holistically interconnected space. To the best of my knowledge, no other artwork—sculptures, pattern designs in woven fabric, pottery, and so on—from the pre-settled era, shows any humanmade borders or geometric designs that demonstrate the concept of framing or dividing space. (There have been some finds of flat painted pebbles with designs such as a cross or a circle with a dot in the center found among some hunting tribes in the period just preceding complex settled life. Such shapes, however, did not find their way into artwork in any substantial way until the pressures of settled life began to be felt.) Such borders and designs seem to have first appeared in various forms of pottery that began to be produced just prior to the advent of high civilizations. At this stage, designs such as the cross (the symbol of quartering) and shapes such as the circle, square, and triangle suddenly appear in various works of art. From this point, almost all works of art were designed with a border, such as a circle or square, creating a circumscribed field that may then have been subdivided by a cross or other geometric patterns.

It simply cannot be the case that prehistoric artists did not have the intelligence or potential brain function to create borders and geometric designs. They had the same brains as later artists, and their mastery of their art form shows high intelligence and a complete grasp of natural forms. Yet their works often overlap, showing a complete lack of regard for the idea of dividing space or formally separating one thing from another. To us today, such art might strike us as sloppy or even childish.

This is because we were taught as children about dividing space and maintaining proportion and how to color "within the lines." Prehistoric artists didn't know about dividing lines because the optical illusion of human consciousness Einstein spoke of had not yet occurred. Their world was a world of overlapping interconnectedness. With such a worldview, the trees of the forest were not clearly separate from the deer, the deer from the bear, or any of these parts from the one observing it all. Even their dreams, as was the case in Chuang Tzu's story, were not clearly separate from the dreamer or the dream state from the waking state.

Like their hunter-gatherer ancestors, modern human babies do not know about the concept of contrasting opposites. We program our children with such concepts when we frame things for them within the relative context of good/bad, boy/girl, right/wrong, big/small, left/right, heavy/light, up/down, and so on. We also teach them about numbers that follow the same format: even/odd, positive/negative, whole/fraction, and how to calculate with numbers via addition and subtraction, multiplication and division. We pass on the concept of countless pairs of opposites, with which borders are created, their contents subdivided, and the parts separated from the whole. Their innocent minds are easily programmed in this manner, as such thinking is all they are exposed to during their formative years.

Virtues of an Uncarved Block

I slowly began to grasp that such concepts are a form of mental programming and not an automatic attribute of the human mind after being exposed to a different manner of thinking in my years of studying Taoist philosophy and spirituality. A primary theme of Taoist philosophy is to encourage one to simplify one's life, especially one's thinking. Students of these teachings learn different methods to restore their original qualities, especially methods to deprogram their minds. Meditative practices are employed to encourage one's mind to settle into a kind of neutral state in which one's programming is not stirred up. Such a neutral state doesn't mean one has no thoughts or emotions but rather that these happen as spontaneous reactions to circumstances, uncolored by preconceived notions of programming.

A good example of the Taoist perspective on this issue of subjective mental programming can be found in chapter 28 of the *Tao Teh Ching*. (For another example of this, see appendix B.) In this teaching, Lao Tzu encourages readers to return to the "absolute integrity of a newborn babe" and the "original simplicity of an uncarved block." He goes on: "When the uncarved block is shaped into useful tools and vessels, its original qualities are destroyed."

The uncarved block Lao Tzu is referring to in this teaching is the objective, natural human mind. He is describing what happens when it is programmed with the subjective system of thought I have been discussing. Perhaps no other teaching more succinctly captures the paradox of ancient Taoist thought than the line referring to the loss of original qualities happening as a result of the gain of useful tools and vessels—another example of the yin/yang seesaw. Many Taoist teachings seem to lament the same changes in technology and cognitive capacity that Western culture hails as representing great advances forward. Taoists believed that their golden era occurred during the countless generations when their hunter-gatherer ancestors lived as one with nature and had innocent minds as pure and unconditioned as an uncarved block. Their only mental programming was that of interconnected nature itself, so they perceived themselves as being truly one with nature, an integral part of the holistically interconnected universe. Eventually, a new mental programming appeared, and while this allowed people to develop useful new technologies, it also caused people to perceive themselves as being separate from their surroundings. They began to see their surroundings as being composed of individual things that were defined by a fixed border and that those things were themselves made up of smaller, individual bits.

Chuang Tzu and other Taoist philosophers proclaimed that this loss of a sense of interconnectedness was the cause of all the problems of civilized life because it spawned feelings of jealousy, competition, and self-centered thinking. If one really believes all people are one, who is there to be jealous of or to compete with? Will one's toes compete with one's fingers or one's liver become jealous of one's spleen? Taoists saw these questions not as mere philosophic puzzles but as the key to understanding the suffering of humanity. When Taoists such as Lao Tzu and Chuang Tzu spoke of this loss of interconnectedness and the value of restoring the mind's original simplicity to be like that of an uncarved block, they did so out of a deep desire to help their fellow beings break through the illusion of individuality—the source of self-centered strife that came to dominate society.

When the subjective mental programming first appeared and the optical illusion within the human consciousness spread, those who would later be called "Taoists" represented a rare breed—the true scientists who understood the utility of the new programming but still objectively perceived all Creation as one. The Taoists responded to this new development by formalizing the yin/yang concepts I have discussed throughout this book. On the surface, these concepts seemed to reinforce or support the new programming—to do as the Romans were doing, so to speak. In actuality, the yin/yang concepts developed by the ancient Taoists contained a subtle but vital twist that was designed to steer people away from the new mental programming and correct the optical illusion in their consciousness. Using a modern analogy, one could even say that the new mental programming was like a computer virus that corrupted the mind's data-processing function and then spread to others, causing most to see themselves and all around them as separate, individual things instead of part of the whole. The Taoists responded by developing a yin/yang antivirus program whose goal was to restore the objective data processing of the human mind. This yin/yang antivirus was applied to the development of many important skills, including the healing arts, in the hope that those who learned and practiced them might have their objectivity restored.

Chinese medicine, along with skills such as martial arts, agricultural, music, and others, was developed with this yin/yang antivirus as its foundation. The reason the concepts of qi, yin/yang, and the five phases seem so mysterious to us today, and even to the Chinese people after the loss of the golden age of innocence, is that they are based on ideas that were developed to counter-program the corrupted way our minds came to process data. To many, these ideas simply do not "compute." It took me years of studying Taoist philosophy under the best possible teacher before I realized that Lao Tzu and other Taoist sages were trying to get the message across that humans were infected with a mental programming virus. It then took even longer for me to understand why they thought that way. Once you understand this point of view, it actually makes a lot of sense, as it has much in common with the way most of us think, save for that one vital twist that makes all the difference in the world. Before I attempt to explain that twist, I will need to dig another layer deeper in deconstructing how the human mind goes about separating the holistically interconnected world around us into individual bits. This may seem difficult to follow at first because most of us do not give much thought to the way our minds go about the job of perception, but please stay with me as I hope my description of this process will eventually begin to make sense to you.

RELATIVE BORDERS

How does the human mind come to designate things as individual? It does this by framing things within a border. It is fairly easy to understand what I mean when I say we frame things within a border when we are considering a three-dimensional object. We might look at a fish, for example, and say it is twelve inches long and two inches wide and three inches deep. Anything beyond that 12x2x3 inches is not the fish. When we say this fish is twelve inches long from its nose to its tail, we are establishing two opposites. The entire length of the fish will be contained between the extreme of the tip of its nose and the opposite extreme of the tip of its tail. The same thing goes with its width and depth—its width is two inches from its right extreme to its left, and its depth is three inches from its top to its bottom. We establish such opposite extremes to help us frame the object and separate it from anything beyond those extremes. If we did not recognize these opposites as constituting the border of the fish, we could not single it out from its surroundings. The yin/yang model, then, helps us frame all three-dimensional objects by establishing the opposite extremes of top/bottom, left/right, and front/back. Once these sets of opposite extremes are established, we can then subdivide between these to single out any smaller part of the whole object. We could say, for example, that the fish's gills are located one quarter of the way (three inches) between its nose and tail. This is what is meant by the term "relative"; we measure a thing in relation to where it is located between a pair of opposite extremes.

Such relative designations or measurements are crucial to Chinese medicine diagnosis. As discussed in chapter 2, a doctor of Chinese medicine tries to establish such things as whether a patient's condition involves too much heat or too much cold, too much moisture or dryness, a qi excess or deficiency, and so on. While measuring in this manner a five-phase version of quartering is often applied, and the patient's condition is classified as hot/warm/neutral/cool/cold, or very moist/slightly moist/neutral/slightly dry/very dry, and so on. Relative measurements such as these are very helpful in breaking down the complex dynamics of a patient's whole being into more manageable bits and seem to support the practice of establishing borders and dividing lines between extremes. But when one considers the laws that underlie Chinese science, the law of opposites, the law of continual change, and so on, as well as the teachings of Lao Tzu, one becomes aware of the vital twist that attempts to deprogram such thinking.

In our fish example, it seems the use of the yin/yang model supports the mental programming that cuts individual things out of the holistically interconnected world around us, circumscribing such things within a framework defined by pairs of opposites. But, if you recall from chapter 1, when I explained the law of opposites holding true across all scales, yin/yang theory holds that while every individual thing is composed of such smaller pair opposites as top/bottom, left/right, and front/back, everything must also be part of a larger yin/yang pairing. So every individual thing such as a fish must itself be part of a larger thing such as the ocean. The ocean itself is a part of the larger earth, the earth part of our solar system, and so on. This twist is also symbolized in the yin/yang symbol, in that it shows the seemingly opposite colors of black and white joined as one, each with a little of its opposite within itself. If black has some white in it, and white has some black, and the two are always joined together, is there truly any such color as black or white? The message of the yin/yang symbol is the heart of the Taoist antivirus program: If we can't separate or even clearly distinguish black from white—are any distinctions real?

THE HEALING POWER OF ACUPRESSURE AND ACUPUNCTURE

The law of opposites and the problems with relative measurements are also an important theme in the first chapter of the *Tao Teh Ching:*

Tao, as the absolute Way of the universe,
*   cannot be conveyed with words.*
That which can be conveyed with words
*   is merely relative conception.*
Although names have been applied to it,
*   the absolute Truth is indescribable.*
One may designate Nothingness
*   as the origin of the universe,*
And Beingness
*   as the mother of the myriad things.*

From the perspective of Nothingness,
*   one may perceive the subtle operation of the universe.*
From the perspective of Beingness,
*   one may distinguish individual things.*
Although differently named, Nothingness and Beingness
*   are one indivisible whole.*
This truth is so subtle.
As the ultimate subtlety,
*   it is the Gate of all Wonders.*

Chapter 1 of the *Tao Teh Ching*, translated by Hua-Ching Ni.

Here Lao Tzu starts by pointing out that all descriptive words convey ideas by describing relative concepts—how something relates to its opposite. Because the Tao encompasses everything—all things and nonthings, all times and timelessness, all space and void—there is nothing other than Tao. As Tao has no opposite to contrast it against, relative descriptions cannot be applied to it. That is why Tao cannot be described with words.

The two primary opposites of nothingness (spirit) and beingness (material) are both contained in Tao. The perspective of nothingness allows one to be aware of the subtle spiritual operation of the universe that connects us all. This was the perspective our early ancestors leaned toward that encouraged the holistic worldview. The perspective of beingness, made popular after the advent of high civilizations, allows one to distinguish individual things such as a fish from the ocean or a dream from a dreamer. This is the perspective modern science is dependent on. The lesson (antivirus twist) of Lao Tzu's first chapter is found in the line in which Lao Tzu says that even the seemingly black and white opposites of material and spiritual are "one indivisible whole." The truth of this fact is so difficult to comprehend (due to the programming virus) that Lao Tzu credits it with being the "Gate of all Wonders." With this teaching, Lao Tzu was downloading the Taoist antivirus.

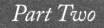

Part Two

SEEKING PROFESSIONAL CARE

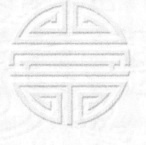

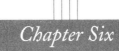

Chapter Six

STRENGTHS AND

WEAKNESSES OF CHINESE

AND WESTERN MEDICINE

Advising modern westerners on how to take advantage of Chinese medicine is somewhat like what a Western health care worker might face trying to educate those in an emerging nation about how to take advantage of Western medicine. Just as Western medicine is a complex mixture of many different practices within one underlying theory of health and disease, so too is Chinese medicine. I have already discussed how the theory of health and disease that underlies Chinese medicine differs from that of Western medicine; I now want to explain some practical details of how to go about using this healing approach that is new to the Western world.

Up to this point I have only discussed acupuncture and acupressure, as these practices are the ones out of the many within the broad umbrella of Chinese medicine that have become most popular here in the West. But offering advice on how to get the most out of Chinese medicine by focusing on acupuncture/acupressure alone would be like the health care worker in the emerging nation focusing only on modern surgery. In addition to acupuncture and acupressure, the use of Chinese herbs is of great importance in Chinese medicine, just as the use of drugs combined with surgery constitutes the cornerstones of Western medicine. By also considering the use of Chinese herbs, we greatly expand our understanding of what Chinese medicine has to offer.

In addition to learning about the strengths and weaknesses of acupuncture/acupressure and Chinese herbs, we should consider something about the training of those delivering those services. When Western medicine is first introduced into an emerging nation, natives there can often obtain drugs and even minor surgery from some well-intended but not fully trained sources. Not only would the health care worker I have been using as an example need to educate locals about how Western medicine views disease and the value of drugs and surgery, they would also need to educate them about whom they should trust to provide those services. The majority of Chinese herbs consumed in the United States are purchased without advice from a professional trained in their use, and acupuncture is preformed by a large number of different health care professionals whose training varies greatly. As Chinese medicine is still in the very early stage of its growth in the United States, with variable standards of training for those who practice it, it will be helpful to review the regulations concerned with its practice, including the training required of the various health care professionals who offer these services.

In the following chapters, then, I will attempt to explain such details as what types of conditions can be treated with Chinese medicine, how many treatments or how much time treatment should take, what results one should expect, how to find qualified practitioners, what risks may be involved, and so on. I will focus on the practices of acupuncture, its close cousin, acupressure, and Chinese herbs. I will also give a brief description of some of the other methods used in Chinese medicine and teach you how to perform some basic acupressure techniques.

To begin this process, I want to take some time putting into perspective the way Chinese medicine works. Over some 20 years of practice, I have conducted thousands of consultations with those who had little understanding of how Chinese medicine works, explaining the nature of the services I provide so that they could make decisions about their treatment options. Of course, when I conduct a consultation, I focus on the specific details of each individual's unique health condition—something I will not be able to do in this format. However, my experience explaining matters to prospective patients has convinced me that once some basic principles are explained and the differences between the therapeutic approaches used in Western and Chinese medicine are put into perspective, most people are then able to make informed decisions about how to integrate Chinese medicine into managing their health care.

The single most important principle one needs to appreciate in order to put these two great medical systems into perspective is to realize that there are two very different approaches that can be employed in treating health disorders. One approach is based on supporting or facilitating the body's ability to heal itself. Most of Chinese medicine and several other so-called alternative medicine systems rely on this approach. The second approach is based on taking over for the body's self-healing ability by directly intervening on a disease (or symptom) process. This is the approach Western medicine is almost completely reliant on. In fact, we in the West have become so dependent on this approach that we have come to believe that it is the only approach possible. This is simply not true. It is possible to base a medical system on facilitating the body's self-healing ability—to help the body to help itself. However, this approach has its own unique characteristics that differ from those of the intervening approach. Understanding these characteristics is essential to learning how to get the most out of either approach alone and how to integrate the two. Because of the different characteristics of these two approaches, I have taken to calling these two "action medicine" and "reaction medicine."

ACTION MEDICINE VS. REACTION MEDICINE

Whenever a healer does something to a patient in an attempt to help the patient's health, the healer is, in effect, taking some sort of action. The healer is manipulating or changing the patient's status quo. When such action is taken, there will be two basic consequences. The first will be the direct consequence of that action, and the second will be the body's reaction to having its status quo changed. To put it simply: every action causes a reaction.

Modern medicine's use of drugs and surgery are examples of action medicine—the intervening approach. When a drug such as an antibiotic is introduced into the body, its direct consequence is to kill bacteria. It will do this in a laboratory petri dish as well as in the human body. Unlike a petri dish, however, when such a substance is introduced into a living system, including the human body, this will also cause some sort of reaction. If this reaction causes harm, it is called a side effect, also known as an adverse reaction. Whether or not the body's reaction to a drug such as an antibiotic causes enough noticeable harm to be called a side effect, there must be some sort of reaction as the body adjusts itself after having its status quo changed.

With action medicine such as drug therapy or surgery, the hope is that the direct consequence of the action will be to improve the patient's problem and that the body's reaction will be minor and of little or no consequence. Acupuncture, on the other hand, is a type of reaction medicine—the self-healing approach. In the case of reaction medicine, the goals are the opposite of those for action medicine—one now hopes the direct action is of little or no consequence and that the reaction will improve the patient's symptoms.

Researchers around the world have been discovering that acupuncture can cause the body to produce a wide array of natural substances, including those that reduce pain and inflammation, enhance immune function, balance hormones, and produce feelings of well-being. The brain imaging research being done by Hang-Zee Cho and others strongly suggests that these effects result from the stimulation of key brain centers that exert control on the body's ability to produce these and other body-regulating substances. This is how reaction medicine works—by stimulating the body to produce its own medicine, as opposed to intervening in place of the body's healing processes, as is done in action medicine. The possibility of stimulating healing reactions is almost completely unknown to modern medicine but actually provides an important complement to action medicine.

As an example of the difference between action and reaction medicine, consider the gardener who wants to control some pests, such as aphids, that are destroying a garden. One method would be to spray the garden with an insecticide that kills aphids. This is usually a pretty reliable way to get rid of the pests, but it can also cause some undesirable effects, such as damaging plants and leaving toxins on plants one may wish to eat. Another method to deal with the problem would be to release ladybugs within the garden or, better yet, grow plants such as dill, cilantro, or caraway that will attract ladybugs to the garden naturally. As aphids are a natural food for ladybugs, having ladybugs in one's garden is a natural way to deal with aphid infestation. The first approach, using insecticide, is similar to what is done in action medicine: employing a manmade agent to intervene on nature. Releasing or attracting ladybugs into the garden is similar to the reaction medicine approach: facilitating nature's own means to control a problem.

Think of the human body as a garden and the bacterial infection as the aphids. Introducing an insecticide into the garden to directly kill the aphids is essentially what happens when antibiotics are used to treat a bacterial infection. Some infections, however, can be successfully treated with acupuncture. In this case, however, the action taken—performing acupuncture on the body—does not directly kill the bacteria but rather stimulates the body's immune response, helping it to do a more effective job of fighting the bacteria itself. This is somewhat like using plants that attract ladybugs to an aphid-infested garden.

Another method that may be used to treat a bacterial infection in Chinese medicine is to use herbs. In the case of Chinese herbs, there is a very wide range of actions. Some herbs are potent substances similar to drugs and work as an action medicine that in this example would directly kill bacteria. Other herbs are very mild substances that work as a reaction medicine by stimulating the body to heal itself. This would be like introducing ladybugs into the garden to eat the aphids. The vast majority of Chinese herbs are of the very mild variety that stimulates the body to heal itself. Many of these herbs have been deemed ineffective when tested by modern researchers because they were tested as though they were action medicine drugs—for example, putting an herb extract in a petri dish with bacteria and then proclaiming it ineffective because the bacteria were not killed. Testing herbs this way is as senseless as placing some acupuncture needles in a petri dish filled with bacteria and then reaching the conclusion that acupuncture is ineffective after the bacteria survive. Reaction medicine works via the body's reaction to a mild stimulus and so can only be studied by observing its effects on real, live subjects.

Another example that can put reaction medicine, especially acupuncture, into perspective is to consider a group of people with mild sinus congestion. One way to treat these people would be to administer antihistamines, an action medicine drug that directly blocks the production of the body's histamine response. The histamine response is a natural function of the body that causes cells to react to allergens, such as sinus cells that produce mucus to flush allergens out of the body. Nature gave us the ability to flush out allergens with the histamine response for good reason. Many of the symptoms we suffer in health problems are part of our body's natural response to the cause of the problem—for example, when our bodies try to flush out an allergen with mucus. A good percentage of action medicine approaches simply short-circuit our body's natural response to a problem. This can make us more comfortable but does nothing to get at the root of the problem.

Imagine, however, that this group with mild sinus congestion could clear it with a good sneeze (I know this is far-fetched, but please play along so that I might make my point). A sneeze is another response the human body has developed over countless generations of evolution to help clear the sinuses. If one were to take a feather and tickle each person in this group under the nostrils, some, perhaps 20 percent or so of this group, would respond by sneezing, thus clearing their congestion. Acupuncture works very much like the feather—it stimulates the body to initiate natural, self-healing responses that nature has endowed us with over millions of years of evolution. Sometimes, for countless reasons, the body is not able to make full use of all the healing resources nature endowed it with. Good reaction medicine helps the body to make better decisions about how to utilize its resources.

I hope these examples have helped to explain these two approaches to healing. Now I can go on to explain some of the characteristics of each approach, as understanding these will help answer many questions about how to utilize Chinese medicine.

In the foregoing example, those who used the action medicine approach of taking antihistamines would probably experience a high rate of relief for their symptoms. Perhaps 70–80 percent of those who took that medicine would experience a reduction in their congestion. However, every action will cause a reaction, and some who took antihistamines will end up with side effects—that is, adverse reactions. The most common of these adverse reactions would be minor things like dryness of the mouth, throat, or sinus. Although it is rare, some who took antihistamines could experience severe reactions such as hallucinations, convulsions, or even cardiovascular collapse.

The point I wish to make here is that the direct consequence of taking action is easy to predict, while the subsequent reactions are difficult to predict. The same will be true when using a feather to cause a sneeze. The direct effect of this action—a slight stimulation of the skin cells touched by the feather—would be largely the same for all the subjects. The number of those who react by sneezing would be much smaller. So here, as in the example of the use of antihistamines, the direct effect of the action was the same for a large percentage of the subjects and thus predictable, while the reaction was much more varied and difficult to predict. Who, exactly, will sneeze when tickled with the feather, and who, exactly, will get what side effect from the antihistamine? Such questions regarding reactions are difficult to answer and thus explain why so many people are seriously harmed by drug side effects; we cannot predict beforehand who will get reactions that are worse than the original problem. If we could predict this, we would not give that drug to those individuals, and drug side effects would not be killing tens of thousands of Americans, as is the case in the United States today.

As action medicine's desired therapeutic effect is a direct result of the action taken, this action must be relatively strong and will thus be relatively easy to predict. That is one of action medicine's greatest strengths. One of its greatest weaknesses, however, is the high rate of undesirable side effects that are much more difficult to predict. In the case of reaction medicine, the desired therapeutic effect takes place as an indirect reaction to the healer's intervention. This intervention will be milder than that used in action medicine, and there will be few if any undesirable effects, but the desired therapeutic effect, being a reaction, will be difficult to predict. Thus, one of the strengths of reaction medicine is its safety, while one of its weaknesses is a relatively greater degree of unpredictability in obtaining the desired therapeutic effect.

The primary strengths and weaknesses of both approaches can be detailed as follows:

ACTION MEDICINE
Strengths
Dramatic results
Faster-acting
Able to save life and limb at critical stages (snatch life out of the jaws of death)
Easier to predict therapeutic outcomes
Easier to study in cause-and-effect manner

REACTION MEDICINE
Strengths
Little or no adverse outcomes
Low-tech and thus low-cost
Treats the cause rather than the symptom
Often causes additional benefits (good side effects)
Able to treat multiple-cause disorders
Can strengthen integrity of body systems and prevent future illness

ACTION MEDICINE
Weaknesses
High rate of difficult-to-predict side effects, including death
Often high-tech and thus high-cost
Treats the symptom more than the cause

REACTION MEDICINE
Weaknesses
More difficult to consistently produce positive outcomes
Often slow-acting (in chronic problems)
Difficult to study in cause-and-effect manner

103

Action Medicine	Reaction Medicine
Weaknesses	**Weaknesses**
Unable to treat multiple-cause disorders	Usually too weak to save life and limb at critical stages
Limited ability to prevent future illness, often causing other illness when prevention is attempted	

Why should it be that the direct consequence of an action is easy to predict, while the inevitable reactions are so difficult to predict? Why is it that the direct consequence of an action like introducing an antihistamine into a human being will largely be the same for all who take that drug, while different people's reactions to this can vary so greatly that doctors are unable to be sure for any given individual that the side effects won't be worse than the original problem? Exploring the answer to this question will further help to clarify the characteristics of action and reaction medicine detailed in the foregoing lists. I believe the answer lies in considering the following question: Are people all the same, or are we all different?

We often hear it said that each person is a unique individual. But is that really true? Nearly all those who took the antihistamine had the same direct consequence—easing of their sinus congestion. If we are all unique individuals, why did taking this action have largely the same direct consequence? The answer, I believe, is that, true to the laws of yin/yang, we are all both the same *and* different at the same time. All of us share traits in common while we also have traits that are very different from one another. Many aspects of human physiology are largely the same for everyone, but as you consider the complete spectrum of human physiology, there are countless variations and subtle differences. Most all of us are born with 10 fingers, yet everyone's fingerprints are unique. One could say the core of the human frame is the same for all, but the fringes, or the in-betweens, vary greatly. The reason the direct consequence of taking action on the body is easy to predict is that this mostly takes place through the core physiology—the aspects we share in common with one another. The reason reactions are so difficult to predict is that these mostly take place through the fringes of our physiology—the subtle, unique variations among us all.

Given that action medicine relies on the traits all people have in common—our "sameness"—action medicine approaches tend to reflect a "one size fits all" mentality. Research is conducted looking for one drug or surgical approach that "works best" for all people with the same disease. Thus, over the last several decades, we have been looking for "a cure" (singular) for cancer or "a cure" for any number of other diseases. If we believed that all people are different, we would realize the "same" disease may happen for different reasons in different people, and we would instead be looking for "different cures" (plural) for these diseases.

Nearly every facet of modern medicine is built upon the assumption that all people are essentially the same. When a doctor orders a lab report such as a blood test, for example, the doctor will get back a computer printout that lists several categories, such as blood glucose or cholesterol levels, and so on. This printout will list the patient's levels for each category, along with what the "normal" range is for each category. Finally, the printout will show if the patient's levels were abnormal—either higher or lower than the normal range. Nowhere on such a list, however, is any consideration given to a patient's individual traits. If we believed individual traits were important, we would try to account for them, realizing, for example, that a low reading for one person may actually be normal for another or a normal reading may actually be abnormal for another. The same thing goes for drug remedies. We look to find the one drug, often even the one dosage of one drug, which will work the best for all people with the same disease.

Whatever unique, individual tendencies people may have, when it comes to diagnosing disorders and prescribing remedies, Western (action) medicine is built upon the notion that individual tendencies can largely be ignored. The one area in which Western medicine acknowledges that unique, individual tendencies impact patient outcomes is when patients develop side effects. In those instances, however, all that is being acknowledged is our inability to predict who may develop what side effect. In other words, the fact that people have unique, individual qualities is not exploited to make action medicine more effective; rather, it is used as an excuse to avoid blame when a patient develops an adverse reaction. When these side effects occur, we are told with a shrug that such reactions are unfortunate but impossible to predict, so no one is really to blame.

The unpredictability of reactions makes reaction medicine difficult to predict also. Because every patient has different qualities and those unique qualities are pivotal to the desired effects of reaction medicine, it is difficult to know how to get the best results for each patient. In the practice of reaction medicine, different approaches may need to be taken to find the best treatment for different people who have the "same" problem, just as one might find one needs to tickle different spots in different people to make them sneeze. This happens frequently in acupuncture, in that acupuncturists often need to try different point combinations before they find those that get the best results. This also happens when prescribing Chinese herbs—several different herb combinations may need to be tried before the best results are obtained.

One of the biggest differences between action and reaction medicine, then, is the manner in which unique, individual tendencies are taken into account. As mentioned earlier, in action medicine, these tendencies are acknowledged but not taken into account in any practical manner. In reaction medicine, individual tendencies are given much more consideration, often proving pivotal to finding the best treatment for each patient. In the practice of Chinese medicine, the individual tendencies that are taken into account are those regarding a person's dynamic state of rising, peaking, and declining qi, as discussed in chapter 2. Two people suffering with migraine headaches, for example, may be found to have different qi imbalances, so the points and/or herbs used in treatment would need to be chosen to address each individual's unique imbalance in order to achieve the best result. Even after an individuals' unique imbalance is determined, different points and herbs may need to be tried. Thus another important difference between action and reaction medicine is that action medicine produces an essentially one-size-fits-all approach to healing while reaction medicine utilizes an array of flexible approaches.

In chapter 3 I mentioned the professor who was frustrated by the holistic theory of interconnectedness and told his class they need not take every falling leaf into account—small influences can be neglected. This is what the modern medicine system ends up doing regarding individual tendencies—it neglects them because they are considered "statistically insignificant." I also explained in that chapter that the holistic theory does not expect us to take every falling leaf into account but does tell us that useful interconnections are so subtle they can be found anywhere—for example, a point on the little toe having a connection with vision. The highly individualized manner in which our bodies react to intervening actions is an example of some of these subtle interconnections. Chinese medicine is largely built on taking these subtle interconnections into account. So while it is true that the unpredictability of reactions makes reaction medicine tricky, as tricky as finding the best spot to tickle with a feather to cause a sneeze, those who are well trained in Chinese medicine are able to take unique, individual tendencies into account and cause desired healing reactions to occur in a good percentage of cases.

MULTIPLE-CAUSE DISORDERS

Because action medicine works by outside intervention—the doctor stepping in and taking over for the body's natural healing ability—another one of its strengths is its ability to deal with acute trauma and even life-threatening situations. In such situations, stimulating the body's self-healing forces with reaction approaches may be too little, too late. You instead need to take more decisive action and take over for the body by directly intervening and changing the status quo. This can be done with surgery, drugs, or radiation therapy or such measures as resetting broken bones, and so on. The very nature of action medicine lends itself to relatively dramatic results, even snatching life out of the jaws of death. Thus one of the strengths and perhaps *the* greatest strength of action medicine is its potential to save life and limb at critical junctures. One of its weaknesses, however, is its less-than-stellar ability to treat a wide range of less immediately critical health problems.

Many of the most stubborn health conditions we face today are those caused by wide-scale breakdowns within multiple body systems. Virtually all of the autoimmune conditions such as multiple sclerosis, rheumatoid arthritis, Crohn's and Graves' disease, psoriasis, fibromyalgia, chronic fatigue syndrome, most neuropathies, certain cancers, a host of degenerative disorders, and many disorders that defy diagnosis are examples of conditions in which many little things go wrong, as opposed to one big thing. In fact, it is quite reasonable to say that we can broadly classify all diseases into two categories: those in which one or a very limited number of big things go wrong and those in which several little things go wrong. While modern medicine has had great success at identifying and dealing with one big problem such as a faulty heart valve, an aggressive bacteria, a broken bone, and so on, it has failed miserably at identifying and dealing with conditions that involve problems in multiple systems.

Chinese medicine, in contrast, is much better suited for dealing with multiple-cause disorders. This is because it is not based on a mechanical cause-and-effect model of nature but one in which disturbances in rising, peaking, and declining qi are measured within a holistically interconnected model of nature. The holistic model assumes that there is an essential interconnection among all parts and thus a disturbance in any part must be felt at some level in every part. The trick is to be able to assess the significant disturbances, especially by ascertaining problems in the patterns of rising, peaking, and declining qi. The next step is to make adjustments by way of a minor action that will cause a reaction in which the whole system adjusts itself. By assuming there is always more than one part involved, the holistic model is much more in its element when dealing with multiple-cause disorders, especially those that are not immediately life-threatening.

Reaction medicine can also be effective in treating single-cause conditions, especially those that are not life-threatening. Acupuncture, acupressure, and Chinese herbs, for example, have a long history of treating martial arts injuries—what we today would call sports injuries. If you sprain a joint or strain a muscle, this is a type of a single-cause disorder that responds well to the aforementioned reaction medicine therapies. In fact, many world-class athletes have discovered that acupuncture can be very effective in treating injuries and improving performance. As effective as these therapies can be for these types of conditions, the majority of people who seek treatment with acupuncture in the United States are those who have tried conventional modern medicine without success. Many of those cases involve multiple-cause disorders. These disorders often take many years to develop and may involve a combination of congenital weaknesses, complications of poor lifestyle habits (poor nutrition, stress, smoking, lack of exercise, etc.), and environmental or other sensitivity/allergy factors. These factors can pile up over years until they reach a critical mass. Modern medicine's focus on finding a singular cause and cure cannot help but fail these conditions, as the only effective treatment involves working on several fronts at the same time, often over many months or even years. A combination of acupuncture/acupressure, diet changes, and herbs, as well as lifestyle modifications, often helps these problems, but progress can be very slow, especially in the beginning stages of treatment.

ADDITIONAL BENEFITS OF
REACTION MEDICINE

In addition to being able to offer hope for multiple-cause disorders, reaction medicine has other strengths in comparison to action medicine. One of the most important and often overlooked strengths of reaction medicine is the potential to provide benefits for problems other than those being treated; that is, to cause good side effects. Because of the nature of holistic interconnections and the fact that reaction medicine takes advantage of these connections in helping the body to help itself, helping one problem with reaction medicine often helps others as well. The very first acupuncture treatment I ever preformed on another person without supervision was one I did on my uncle for his tennis elbow while I was still in acupuncture school. A few days after this treatment, he called me and asked if I had also done something to treat his chronic constipation because this had cleared up along with his arm pain. The truth was, I did not even know he had constipation, but the point I used to treat his tennis elbow was on the large intestine qi pathway, and that point is often used to treat constipation.

Finding that other health conditions improve in the process of treating the primary problem is a common occurrence in the practice of Chinese medicine. Often these additional benefits go unnoticed by the patient at first. Because reaction medicine helps the body to better adjust and heal itself naturally, many people do not realize that the cause of their sleeping better, catching fewer colds, experiencing more energy, and so on is the treatment they have been having for other problems. If someone continues to be treated with reaction medicine approaches over longer periods of time, the improvements in overall body balancing they experience can also help to prevent future health problems. This fact is difficult to convince modern skeptics of as it is difficult to prove that doing something over extended periods of time will prevent problems in the distant future. The Chinese were able to learn this about herbs, dietary intake, acupuncture/acupressure treatments, exercises like tai chi and qi-gong, and so on, only after observing many generations of people utilizing these practices. When a family or certain school of thought, for example, would develop a new herb formula or exercise style, people could then see the results of these practices over generations. If those undertaking such practices experienced better health, it became obvious to those in their community, since much of life in China historically took place in simple towns and villages, where life stayed largely the same over literally centuries of time.

Action medicine, in contrast, has had much less success in preventing future illness. While it is true that one of the greatest accomplishments of modern medicine has been controlling many of the world's worst infectious diseases by developing vaccinations and inoculations, these approaches are actually modern medicine's exception to its dependence on action medicine. If you think about it, inoculations are actually a type of reaction medicine. A very minor type of action is taken on the body (introduction of the inoculation agent) but this action is not the desired therapy. The desired therapy comes as a result of the body's natural *reaction* to the initial action, in this case, the production of antibodies to a certain pathogen that allows the immune system to more rapidly respond to an invasion of this pathogen in the future.

When true action medicine approaches are used in an attempt to prevent future disorders, the old problem of undesirable side effects come into play. This was recently seen in the case of the major study on hormone replacement therapy (HRT). Researchers were hoping to show that women who took HRT would have less risk of heart disease. Instead they found that HRT actually caused an increased risk of heart disease and breast cancer, as well as increased incidence of blood clots and stroke. Millions of women had been taking HRT for decades, especially for the prevention of osteoporosis (brittle bones) as well as to control menopausal symptoms. I do not know if anyone has yet tried to calculate how many women suffered strokes, blood clots, or heart disease or contracted breast cancer because they had been prescribed HRT to reduce menopausal symptoms or help reduce the risk of osteoporosis or heart disease. Such side effects are especially unacceptable when you consider that there are safer reaction medicine therapies that can treat such problems.

Chapter Seven

ANSWERING COMMON

QUESTIONS ABOUT

TREATMENT

Now THAT I HAVE EXPLAINED THE strengths and weaknesses of action and reaction approaches, I can more easily address the most common questions people have about the use of acupuncture and the other therapies used in Chinese medicine. It is important to keep in mind that Chinese medicine consists of several different therapies, acupuncture/acupressure and herbs being the most fundamental but not the only approaches that may be used. I like to think of the various techniques used in Chinese medicine as different tools. When treating any given problem, the healer may be able to deal with that problem by using only one tool but might just as easily find he or she needs to use some of the other tools. This can vary from person to person, even those with the "same" problem. Some may respond well to one technique (tool); another person with the same problem might respond better with another technique. For example, one person with asthma may respond well to acupuncture alone, another may only respond to herbs, and a third might require both of those therapies and to also practice breathing exercises. As already mentioned, contrary to the one-size-fits-all approach of Western medicine, the use of reaction therapies like those in Chinese medicine often requires a lot of flexibility in finding the best approach to treat any given individual.

Each of the techniques listed hereafter may be applied alone and be performed by a specialist who only practices that one method, or they may be used in combination, either by a team approach employing different specialists or by someone trained to perform multiple techniques. While some techniques such as acupuncture or acupressure are very similar and thus can be used to treat similar conditions, each type of therapy has its own characteristics, making them relatively more or less suited for treating different specific conditions.

VARIOUS TECHNIQUES OF CHINESE MEDICINE

Acupuncture: Insertion of fine needles into specific spots throughout the body to help the body to heal a wide range of disorders.

Electro-acupuncture: A mild electrical current is administered through acupuncture needles, usually by attaching wires from an electrical stimulating device to the handles of the acupuncture needles with small clips. Stimulation may be applied with electrodes attached directly to the acupuncture points without the use of needles, although technically this is not a form of acupuncture because the skin is not pierced.

Acupressure: Similar to acupuncture, in that "acu" points are stimulated to balance qi and help a wide range of disorders, although the skin is not pierced.

Chinese herbal medicine: Although the term "herbs" or "herbal" is used, this form of therapy includes substances from plant, animal, and mineral sources. Internal varieties may be given in pill, powder, liquid, including liquid extract, form or in the form of raw, dried ingredients that are decocted (boiled) as teas. Topical herbal remedies can be applied as liquids, creams, powders, or plasters that attach to the skin.

Moxibustion: Various methods of burning a specific herb known as "moxa" (*Artemisia vulgaris*) either at specific points or over a larger area. Originally developed in northern China as a method to combat "invasion of cold," moxa is now used for treating a variety of problems.

Chinese nutrition or food therapy: A unique system of using foods based on yin/yang and five phase models rather than modern notions of the chemical composition (vitamin/mineral content, etc.) of foods.

Exercise therapies: Various exercises, the most popular of these being tai chi chuan, qi-gong (chi-gong), and breathing exercises. All of these are also based on yin/yang, five phase principles.

Qi-gong: Also known as medical qi-gong, this is the most subtle of all Chinese medicine therapies in which the therapist uses his or her own qi to influence the qi of the patient, sometimes without physical touch.

Oriental massage techniques, including tui-na: A wide range of massage, pressure, and manipulation techniques, some of which are similar to what we would call physical therapy in the West.

Cupping: A method of using glass, plastic, or bamboo cups to enhance circulation. A vacuum is created inside the cup, and then it is placed on the skin. The suction inside the cups slightly raises the skin, and then the cups are usually moved around. Most commonly used for various muscular pains or in treating colds or flu.

Bleeding techniques: Used in conjunction with acupuncture, very small amounts of blood are extracted, often just a few drops after a very superficial puncture. Used to release heat or help to resolve stagnant blood within a muscle. This technique is nothing like the copious bleeding therapy used in prescientific Western medicine.

Gwa sa: A technique similar in function to cupping and involving various methods of lightly scraping the skin to enhance circulation and draw out "blood impurities." In Asia, this is a widely used folk technique, especially on children. As a certain type of large coin is sometimes used, this technique is also known as "coining."

When wondering what conditions can be treated with Chinese medicine, one factor to consider is the training of the healer and especially how many tools he or she may be able to draw upon to treat different conditions. One trained in acupuncture alone may not be as effective as one equally trained in acupuncture but also in the use of some of Chinese medicine's other tools. Another factor to consider is the question of what tools a patient is willing to let the healer use in the treatment and also what self-care the patient is willing to do. Will the person who goes to an acupuncturist be willing to take herbs or practice breathing exercises? There is an old saying popular among doctors of Chinese medicine: "You can write an herbal prescription for someone, but you can't drink the tea for them." Those seeking help must share in the responsibility of their treatment, especially in reaction medicine approaches that attempt to heal problems naturally. The answer to the question of what conditions can be successfully treated with Chinese medicine, then, rests partly in the question of how fully a person is willing to cooperate in the treatment.

I just gave you a brief description of the more common treatment methods used in Chinese medicine. The vast majority of these approaches are types of reaction medicine therapies and so work to help the body to heal itself as is the case with acupuncture. Many licensed acupuncturists will have learned to utilize at least some of these additional techniques. Most of the other health care professionals who practice acupuncture have learned that technique as a supplement to their primary Western medicine training and rarely learn to use the additional tools available in Chinese medicine (although they have

learned to use other Western medicine tools). I will consider the training of the various health care professionals who use some form of
Chinese medicine techniques in the next chapter.

CONDITIONS THAT CAN BE TREATED
WITH CHINESE MEDICINE

As discussed in the last chapter, action and reaction therapies have different strengths and weaknesses, including the types of conditions
they can treat. Reaction medicine helps the body to heal itself and so
works best for problems the body has the potential to heal. Action
medicine works best for problems the body does not have the potential to heal. If you were to dislocate your shoulder joint, for example,
you could not treat it by stimulating the body's self-healing ability
alone. You would need to take action and physically manipulate the
joint back into place. If your shoulder joint were to become inflamed,
however, this could be treated with reaction medicine, as the body has
the ability to fight inflammation. Thus, when wondering what types of
conditions can be treated with reaction medicine such as acupuncture
and most of the rest of Chinese medicine, one should consider whether
the condition can or cannot be healed by the body's self-healing ability. Of course, this is not always a simple question to answer, as there
are many factors that will determine this.

The World Health Organization (WHO) has done a lot of work
in the area of traditional medical approaches of various cultures. They
recognized that acupuncture is spreading rapidly around the world
and so gave special consideration to advising countries how they may
come to understand the training necessary to become a qualified
acupuncturist and the types of conditions that are treatable. While
saying that it is up to each national health authority to decide what
conditions they wish to use acupuncture to treat, the WHO provided

a rough guideline by compiling a comprehensive list of controlled clinical trials done on acupuncture and then dividing these findings into four categories. These categories cover a span from those conditions for which acupuncture has been clearly proven effective to those conditions for which fewer studies have been done but evidence suggests acupuncture may be worthwhile trying.

A review of these four categories shows that, as a general rule, those conditions that acupuncture has more clearly shown itself effective in treating are largely conditions that readily respond to the body's self-healing ability. Conversely, the conditions for which acupuncture's effectiveness is less certain tend to be of the type for which the body's self-healing ability alone may not be effective. The first list is thus dominated by conditions such as hay fever, headache, low back pain, morning sickness, and tennis elbow—conditions the body clearly has the ability to heal. In the second list we start to find more conditions for which the body's ability to heal itself is less certain, such as bronchial asthma, infertility, and chronic ulcerative colitis. The last two lists are made up of conditions like color blindness, deafness, and chronic pulmonary heart disease, and then coma, convulsions, and viral encephalitis. These last conditions are good examples of those that the body's self-healing ability could *possibly* address but for which the odds of this happening are considerably less than for the disorders on the first two lists. One category not listed by the WHO is those conditions for which acupuncture is clearly not effective. Such a list would be dominated by conditions that require action medicine such as severe trauma, aggressive infections, badly degenerated joints, congenital disorders, or a range of near-fatal conditions. When I say acupuncture would not be effective in treating these conditions, though, I mean as a primary treatment meant to cure or control such problems. Acupuncture or other reaction therapies can be quite helpful as a supplemental therapy in such conditions to ease pain, speed recovery, or otherwise improve general well-being.

Although these lists only reflect conditions for which controlled trials on acupuncture have been done and cannot cover every possible condition, a review of these lists gives a good general sense of the types of conditions that are most treatable with acupuncture. The WHO's lists, as given on their website under "Acupuncture: Review and analysis of reports on controlled clinical trials," are as follows.

DISEASES AND DISORDERS THAT CAN BE TREATED WITH ACUPUNCTURE

The diseases or disorders for which acupuncture therapy has been tested in controlled clinical trials reported in the recent literature can be classified into four categories, as shown below.

1. Diseases, symptoms, or conditions for which acupuncture has been proved—through controlled trials—to be an effective treatment:

Adverse reactions to radiotherapy and/or chemotherapy

Allergic rhinitis (including hay fever)

Biliary colic

Depression (including depressive neurosis and depression following stroke)

Dysentery, acute bacillary

Dysmenorrhea, primary

Epigastralgia, acute (in peptic ulcer, acute and chronic gastritis, and gastrospasm)

Facial pain (including craniomandibular disorders)

Headache

Hypertension, essential

Hypotension, primary

Induction of labor

Knee pain

Leukopenia

Low back pain

Malposition of fetus, correction of

Morning sickness

Nausea and vomiting

Neck pain

Pain in dentistry (including dental pain and
temporomandibular dysfunction)

Periarthritis of shoulder

Postoperative pain

Renal colic

Rheumatoid arthritis

Sciatica

Sprain

Stroke

Tennis elbow

2. Diseases, symptoms, or conditions for which the therapeutic effect of acupuncture has been shown but for which further proof is needed:

Abdominal pain (in acute gastroenteritis or due to
gastrointestinal spasm)

Acne vulgaris

Alcohol dependence and detoxification

Bell's palsy

Bronchial asthma

Cancer pain

Cardiac neurosis

Cholecystitis, chronic, with acute exacerbation

Cholelithiasis

Competition stress syndrome

Craniocerebral injury, closed

Diabetes mellitus, non-insulin-dependent

Earache

Epidemic hemorrhagic fever

Epistaxis, simple (without generalized or local disease)

Eye pain due to subconjunctival injection

Facial spasm

Female infertility

Female urethral syndrome

Fibromyalgia and fasciitis

Gastrokinetic disturbance

Gouty arthritis

Hepatitis B virus carrier status

Herpes zoster (human [alpha] herpesvirus 3)

Hyperlipemia

Hypo-ovarianism

Insomnia

Labor pain

Lactation, deficiency

Male sexual dysfunction, nonorganic

Ménière's disease

Neuralgia, postherpetic

Neurodermatitis

Obesity

Opium, cocaine, and heroin dependence

Osteoarthritis

Pain due to endoscopic examination

Pain in thromboangiitis obliterans

Polycystic ovary syndrome (Stein-Leventhal syndrome)

Postextubation in children

Postoperative convalescence

Premenstrual syndrome

Prostatitis, chronic

Pruritus

Radicular and pseudoradicular pain syndrome

Raynaud syndrome, primary

Recurrent lower urinary tract infection

Reflex sympathetic dystrophy

Retention of urine, traumatic

Schizophrenia

Sialism, drug-induced

Sjögren syndrome

Sore throat (including tonsillitis)

Spine pain, acute

Stiff neck

Temporomandibular joint dysfunction

Tietze syndrome

Tobacco dependence

Tourette syndrome

Ulcerative colitis, chronic

Urolithiasis

Vascular dementia

Whooping cough (pertussis)

3. Diseases, symptoms, or conditions for which there are only individual controlled trials reporting some therapeutic effects, but for which acupuncture is worth trying because treatment by conventional and other therapies is difficult:

Chloasma

Choroidopathy, central serous

Color blindness

Deafness

Hypophrenia

Irritable colon syndrome

Neuropathic bladder in spinal cord injury
Pulmonary heart disease, chronic
Small airway obstruction

4. Diseases, symptoms, or conditions for which acupuncture may be tried, provided the practitioner has special modern medical knowledge and adequate monitoring equipment:
Breathlessness in chronic obstructive pulmonary disease
Coma
Convulsions in infants
Coronary heart disease (angina pectoris)
Diarrhea in infants and young children
Encephalitis, viral, in children, late stage
Paralysis, progressive bulbar and pseudobulbar

DISTINGUISHING WHAT CAN AND CAN'T BE SELF-HEALED

Much of what I do when someone comes to me for an initial consultation is to consider a wide range of information to determine what the odds are that the therapies I provide will be effective for them. What I am really trying to figure out is whether or not their condition will respond to reaction medicine's effect of helping the body's self-healing ability to reach its full potential. Unfortunately, I cannot always be sure of this by determining whether their condition is of the variety that the body can heal. While it is true that reaction medicine should be able to help those conditions that can be healed by the body's innate healing abilities, there are exceptions. Consider for example, a diabetic who has a small cut on the foot. In most all circumstances, a small cut on the foot can be healed by the body's self-healing ability and would be helped to do this faster by the right kind of reaction medicine such as acupuncture. Many diabetics, however, have great difficulty healing cuts or other wounds, especially in their lower extremities. This is because their disease can adversely affect a wide range of body processes, including reducing circulation in the lower extremities. It is tragic that for some diabetics, a small cut or sore on their lower extremities can fester, leading to gangrene that may require the afflicted limb to be amputated.

Can a reaction therapy such as acupuncture, that normally works so well to help heal a cut, help a nonhealing cut on the foot of a diabetic? The answer is that it might, but then again it might not. Acupuncture should consistently be able to help a diabetic's self-healing efforts to be more effective, but it can be difficult to know in any given case if the help this brings will be enough to make the critical difference. Many health problems will have a critical threshold that makes all the difference in the world. On the wrong side of this threshold the problem lingers, on the other side of this threshold the body's healing efforts get the upper hand and resolve the problem. Some diabetics with a cut on the foot may be so far below this critical threshold that the improvement in the body's self-healing efforts acupuncture causes will not be enough to get over the hump and heal the problem. In other cases, the help from reaction medicine will push things over this threshold and give the body's self-healing efforts the upper hand, thus healing the problem.

How does one tell if a problem is near enough to the critical threshold and likely to be helped by reaction medicine or if it is too far gone? There are many signs we look for in Chinese medicine to help us determine how far out of balance a patient may be, but even without such specialized training there are some common sense things to consider to help people get an idea of what the odds are that their problem may respond to reaction medicine. For example, what is the person's overall health status, age, and so on? Using the diabetes example again, a diabetic with a foot sore who is in relatively good overall health will have a better chance to improve than one whose overall health is poor—perhaps troubled by other health problems—or is badly overweight, and so on. A younger person at the same level of health as an older one is likely to do better, but if the older one is in better overall health they may do better than the younger one.

Considering all the foregoing, then, when wondering what health problems can be treated with acupuncture and the rest of Chinese medicine, one needs to consider if the problem is a type that has the potential to be healed with the body's self-healing efforts. Next, one needs to consider many aspects of the patient's overall heath; age, weight, use of prescription medications, and so on. Are they willing to follow advice about exercise, or taking herbs to improve their chances for recovery? Finally, what about the training of the healer? How many tools does he or she have available, and what is his or her level of expertise with any given tool? In the real world of health care, it is often more a matter of whether a particular person with a health problem can be helped by a particular healer than whether a certain disease can be treated with a particular type of therapy. A health care professional who is well trained in acupuncture or other reaction therapy should be able to help determine the odds of success on the basis of these and other factors.

How Many Treatments Might Be Needed?

In addition to wanting to know what types of problems can be treated with Chinese medicine, people will also want to know how many treatments or how long a period of treatment will be needed. Because Chinese medicine is almost exclusively a method of reaction medicine and this approach differs so much from individual to individual, answering this question is also difficult. Some of the factors I discussed earlier in addressing what types of conditions can be treated also apply here: the age of the patient, overall health, and so on.

As a general rule, the longer someone has had a problem, the longer it will take to treat. Fortunately, this does not mean it takes exactly as long to treat as it took to develop the problem. I tell my patients that if a problem took years to develop, it may take months to treat, a problem that took months to develop will usually take weeks to treat, one that took weeks to develop may only take days to treat, and something that just popped up may resolve in just one or two treatments.

As far as acupuncture and acupressure go, treatments are usually begun at a more frequent pace, perhaps two or three treatments per week, before the frequency is reduced to once a week or once every other week. In some acute conditions, it is often useful to do a few daily treatments to get the problem under control before spreading the treatments out. The frequency of the treatments is dictated more by cost than by therapeutic value. While the Chinese are now beginning to move away from fully socialized medicine, over the last few decades many medical services were provided at no cost. In such a system, acupuncture was often done daily, perhaps for 10 days in a row. This was called a "series" of treatments. Some patients would undergo several series of treatments. In the United States, while there is some insurance coverage for acupuncture, many patients have to pay out-of-pocket for treatment. Due to these cost concerns, many acupuncturists have learned how to squeeze the most benefit out of the least number of treatments by spacing them out, as mentioned earlier. If one can afford it, it is better to do more frequent treatment, as this can speed recovery.

I like to tell those under my care that every treatment process will have a beginning, a middle, and an ending phase. The beginning phase consists of making something positive happen for them; the middle is where you build on that progress and take the improvement as far as possible. The last phase is making the improvement last as long as possible. Although every person is different and can respond differently to treatment, those who get off to a faster start and show more improvement sooner in the first phase will almost always end up needing fewer treatments overall than those who take longer before they first see any improvement. Because of this, I often tell people that I will be able to advise them how many treatments will end up being needed only after I see how well they respond in the first phase. In complex cases, I often recommend five to eight treatments over three to five weeks as a good first phase. Most people should show some progress during this time, and then, depending on the degree of progress, I will be able to tell them how many more treatments are likely to be necessary in total. Some people will have significant improvement within the first one or two treatments and may only require a few more treatments after that, especially if their problem is a more recent one. Complex or chronic problems may only begin to respond after five to six treatments.

However many treatments it takes before symptoms begin to improve, once improvement begins and one moves into the second phase of treatment, this improvement should build over time. This may not happen with each and every treatment, but progress should be steady overall. This phase is like watching a graph chart of the stock market: there may be a dip one day, but overall you want to see steady improvement. Eventually this improvement will plateau, either with the elimination of all symptoms or with only partial improvement. If the improvement is only partial, it is possible that more treatment will once again move things beyond this plateau and provide further improvement. Knowing if the treatment has reached its maximum therapeutic value or is just at a temporary plateau is one of the more difficult things in reaction medicine. Sometimes it is wise to take a short break from treatment, perhaps two or three weeks, before starting another round of treatments, as this can help jump-start the progress again.

Once the maximum therapeutic value of the treatment has been reached, the final phases of treatment consist of doing a few more treatments with longer periods of time between, perhaps, two to four weeks. This is done to see if the improvement holds or if the symptoms start to return. If symptoms return, then the last phase had not been reached, and more treatment is needed. If there is no return of the symptoms, then treatment can be suspended, and the problem should not return. People often ask if the effects of acupuncture are temporary. They should not be, unless some significant stress on the affected area that was treated occurs. For example, if someone has suffered low back pain for ten years and goes through three months of treatment in which the pain completely resolves, the pain should not return two weeks, or even two months, after treatment is stopped. If, in this example, this patient should have a fall a year or two later and land on the back, they might again develop back pain, but otherwise the original problem should have been healed, as reaction medicine helps the body to heal itself.

Chapter Eight

HOW TO FIND A

QUALIFED PRACTITIONER

I MENTIONED IN THE PREVIOUS chapter that the real question is often not so much whether a type of therapy can treat a specific disease but whether or not an individual with a certain health disorder can be helped by an individual healer. More than anything, providing health care is really about people helping people. While the type of approach—the particular action medicine or reaction medicine—is certainly important, the training, experience, and degree of caring an individual provider brings to the healer-patient relationship is just as important.

In this chapter I will do my best to give you advice about how to find qualified providers of the primary therapies used in Chinese medicine. Of course, no such advice can carry with it a guarantee that these health care providers will be the answer for every person's problems.

However, knowing some facts about the training different health care providers undergo can be helpful in making decisions when choosing to pursue their services. The section on acupuncturists is divided into two parts, as the regulations regarding the practice of acupuncture are complex.

How to Find a Qualified Acupuncturist

Since first bursting on the U.S. health care scene in the early 1970s, the practice of acupuncture has grown rapidly, spawning the birth of a new healing profession and finding its way into the practice of several already established fields of health care. It is not legal for anyone in the United States to perform acupuncture unless they hold some sort of licensing or certification. However, these laws vary considerably from state to state, making it difficult for consumers to make informed choices about how to seek out providers of acupuncture therapy.

If we elect to call any health care professional who sticks acupuncture needles in people an "acupuncturist," then we can say the education range of different acupuncturists in the United States covers everything from those who went through thousands of hours of training over years of time, passed rigorous examinations, and have had decades of experience treating tens of thousands of patients to those who have no formal training, have never passed any examinations, have little experience, and practice part-time on a very limited number and type of patients. You may be surprised to learn that most, but not all, states allow medical doctors and osteopaths to practice acupuncture without requiring them to undergo any formal training or examination in that subject. Some states allow chiropractors or naturopaths to perform acupuncture with some training but no required examination. Still other states allow podiatrists, dentists, physician's assistants, nurses, or even drug detox specialists to perform acupuncture in some restricted manner, some of these without any required formal education or examinations.

At the other end of the spectrum are health care professionals whose training and practice are based upon acupuncture and Chinese medicine, and they are usually titled as a licensed or certified acupuncturist. Most, but not all, states have laws authorizing acupuncture to be performed by a licensed/certified acupuncturist. At the time of my writing this chapter, forty states and the District of Columbia have such laws (practice acts). All of these licensed/certified acupuncturists were required to have completed an accredited educational program and pass formal examinations. (Before the first formal education and examination programs were established in the United States, the very first licensed/certified acupuncturists here were granted this title or "grandfathered," based on proof of their previous experience. These were few in number, and most had years of experience practicing in the Far East.) Ten states—Alabama, Delaware, Kansas, Kentucky, North Dakota, Mississippi, Michigan, Oklahoma, South Dakota, and Wyoming—have no regulations allowing specialists to practice acupuncture, although most of these states allow medical doctors, osteopaths, or chiropractors, and perhaps others, to perform acupuncture. I will discuss the maze of acupuncture regulations later in this section; the point I wish to stress here is that there is a very wide range of training and experience among the various health care professionals who practice acupuncture.

Licensed/certified acupuncturists constitute what I will from this point refer to as the "acupuncture profession," meaning those whose medical practice is primarily based around the practice of acupuncture. I use this term to distinguish those professionals from others who practice acupuncture as an adjunct to their primary practice and licensing, such as chiropractic, naturopathic, or allopathic (Western) medicine. As you might imagine, many of those in the acupuncture profession believe that they are the most qualified acupuncturists, as that practice is their "main thing," as opposed to other health care providers who have less formal training in acupuncture, have not been required to pass formal acupuncture exams in order to practice, and only use acupuncture to supplement the primary health care system they were originally trained in. On the other hand, many chiropractors, naturopaths, osteopaths, and medical doctors believe their training in acupuncture makes them at least equally qualified to perform that service while their training in their primary field makes them a more well-rounded health care provider.

Unfortunately, these different groups have not had especially cordial relationships between them regarding the issue of acupuncture training and practice. At one extreme are some in the acupuncture profession who strongly believe that only those formally educated and licensed by passing state approved licensing/certification exams in acupuncture should be allowed to perform that service. At the other extreme are some medical doctors who believe that licensed/certified acupuncturists do not have enough training in Western medicine and so should only practice under the supervision of medical doctors. For the most part, however, neither extreme prevails, as most states (but not all) allow licensed/certified acupuncturists to practice without M.D. supervision or referral, while allowing other health care professionals to practice acupuncture without requiring them to take full, accredited acupuncture training and examinations.

Where does this leave the average consumer who is interested in pursuing acupuncture but is confused about whether to seek a licensed/certified acupuncturist or an M.D., D.O., D.C, or N.D. who performs acupuncture? While there is more variation in formal training among those who practice acupuncture than in most other health care fields, consumers seeking acupuncture treatment should carry out the same commonsense investigation one would do when looking for a "good" doctor or surgeon. After first verifying that the acupuncture provider has undergone the training required to legally practice (I will go over these requirements a little later), you should ask the same kinds of questions you would ask any professional you are considering entrusting with your care. How much experience have they had in treating similar medical problems? How many treatments do they think it will take before improvements should be seen or until the treatment process is finished? How much will each treatment cost? Will insurance cover any of the cost—if so, how much? In addition to these general questions, you should also ask if disposable needles will be used. If needles are reused, ask how they will be sterilized. Some states require licensed/certified acupuncturists to use only disposable needles (most acupuncturists use these anyway), but all states require anyone doing acupuncture to use properly sterilized equipment.

As with any health care provider, those providing acupuncture should be able to answer these questions to your satisfaction. However, one should also follow one's gut feelings. In addition to the specific answers you get to these questions, consider your instincts. Did you feel comfortable with your encounter with this health care provider? Did anything about them rub you the wrong way? While it may be true that the specific mechanisms of acupuncture remain a mystery, those performing acupuncture should not seem mysterious themselves and should act in a professional manner. While some may explain that acupuncture treats the body/mind/spirit in a holistic fashion, these professionals are trained and licensed to provide a medical service, not a spiritual or religious service. This is an extreme example to make my point: if you are seeking treatment for tennis elbow and are told the problem is bad karma from a past life and you need to undergo a spiritual ceremony to treat it, such a diagnosis and prescription would be as out of the realm of normal practice for anyone providing acupuncture as it would be for Western medicine treatment from a medical doctor. If you feel uncomfortable with your encounter in any way— find someone else to treat you.

As for my personal opinion of the qualifications of licensed/certified acupuncturist versus those other health care professionals who perform acupuncture—as I am a licensed acupuncturist, my first instinct is to support the notion that those who make this practice their main specialty are the most qualified. However, as I have gotten to know some in other health care fields who practice acupuncture, I have been impressed to find that there are some medical doctors, osteopaths, chiropractors, naturopaths, and so on who have developed a love for acupuncture and have gone far beyond the limited training their states require to legally practice. While it is true that, as a general rule, licensed/certified acupuncturists undergo more required training and take the subject of acupuncture more seriously than other health care professionals, this does not mean that all licensed/certified acupuncturists are necessarily more qualified than everyone else. True to the laws of yin/yang, there are always exceptions to the general rule; a little white in the black and a little black in the white. Consumers would be wise to watch for those exceptions—supposedly well-trained licensed/certified acupuncturists who fall short of the level of competency normally found in their profession, and those other acupuncture providers who have gone above and beyond their limited required training and exceed the average level of competency of most part-time acupuncturists.

The good news about acupuncture is that, as a general rule, the procedure is very safe—much more so on average than many conventional Western medical approaches. I will discuss the risks of acupuncture later in this chapter; the reason I mention acupuncture's relative safety here is to suggest that the main problem with being treated by someone who is not thoroughly trained in acupuncture is not so much that they may do you some harm but that they will be less likely to do you any good. In chapter 6 I described acupuncture as a type of reaction medicine that can be as tricky to make work as trying to make someone sneeze by tickling their nose with a feather. Those with the most training and experience in nose tickling will cause a higher percentage of people to sneeze than those with less training and experience, but neither one will cause harm trying. Of course, acupuncture does carry more risk than tickling a nose with a feather, but my bottom line here is that, due to acupuncture's relative safety, I cannot honestly tell you that you should never consider getting acupuncture from anyone who is not a fully trained, licensed/certified acupuncturist. If you have the option, it makes sense to seek out those with the higher level of training, but, in addition to those states that don't have practice acts legally recognizing licensed/certified acupuncturists, several states have a very limited number of those specialists. Some seeking acupuncture services may find their only resource for those services to be from those other health care fields. Whatever the situation, I would recommend that, in addition to the commonsense advice I gave you earlier, just keep in mind that if you are being treated with acupuncture and are not being helped for your problem, this does not necessarily mean that acupuncture cannot help you. It may be that the person doing the treatment is just not knowledgeable enough to make acupuncture work for you and that someone else with more ability could. This is especially true if your condition is one that is likely to respond to acupuncture, as discussed in the last chapter.

REGULATIONS FOR PRACTICE AS A LICENSED/CERTIFIED ACUPUNCTURIST

In addition to the different regulations for practicing acupuncture between the different health care professions, there are, in essence, two different sets of regulations for those in the acupuncture profession. Thirty-nine of the forty states that license acupuncturists follow one set of regulations while one state, my state of California, follows another. California has its own system for establishing education requirements, accrediting schools, and overseeing a licensing examination process. Those completing this process will be designated a licensed acupuncturist with the initials L.Ac. Almost all the other states require acupuncture specialists to have taken the exams of and/or obtained certification from an organization known as the National Certification Commission for Acupuncture and Oriental Medicine (NCCAOM). Those with that certification will have been granted the title of a diplomate in acupuncture, designated by the initials Dip.Ac. (NCCAOM). Even with that certification and those initials, different states then grant titles such as licensed acupuncturist (L.Ac. or Lic.Ac.), certified acupuncturist (C.A.), or registered acupuncturist (R.Ac.). Four states grant titles with wording including the term "doctor" or "physician," as in "doctor of oriental medicine" or "acupuncture physician." Unfortunately, California, which accounts for more than one-third of all U.S. acupuncture specialists, does not recognize NCCAOM certification, and only around ten of the thirty-nine other states leave open the option of recognizing California's acupuncture licensing.

To become a licensed acupuncturist in California, one must pass two state examinations. In order to qualify to take those examinations, one must graduate from a state-approved instruction program. Most meet this requirement by graduating from a state-approved acupuncture school that teaches the courses required by the state. Starting January 1, 2005, these schools will be required to teach a minimum of 3,000 hours, an increase from the 2,348 hours that had been previously required. The training for California licensed acupuncturists includes basic Western sciences and Western medicine training as well as acupuncture and oriental medical subjects such as Chinese herbal medicine. The two other routes of eligibility to take the California acupuncture exams are completing an approved tutorial program or an approved foreign training program. Both the tutorial and foreign training programs must meet or surpass the requirements of the state-approved schools.

As already mentioned, most other states that license/certify acupuncturists require passage of the examinations of the NCCAOM. As in California, to take these examinations, one must meet education requirements set by the NCCAOM. These include completion of a training program in an approved acupuncture school, including some foreign schools; apprenticeship; or a combination of those two. Unlike the California Acupuncture Board, which sets education standards and approves schools, in addition to administering their exams, the NCCAOM develops and administers their exams but the standards of training and approval of schools is done by another organization, the Accreditation Commission for Acupuncture and Oriental Medicine (ACAOM), an organization approved by the U.S. Department of Education to accredit acupuncture training programs. Like California, the ACAOM recently increased its standards for the hours required to complete its approved training in acupuncture and Chinese herbs. They now require their accredited schools to teach at least 1,905 hours (up from 1,725 previously required) for acupuncture programs that do not include Chinese herbs and 2,625 hours (up from 2,175 previously required) for those programs that include Chinese herbs.

The recent rise in training hours by ACAOM and the state of California are a reflection of the trend to increase educational standards as the acupuncture profession matures. A major issue within the acupuncture profession is the question of how much Western medicine acupuncturists should be required to learn. In China and Korea, those learning acupuncture in the medical schools get extensive training in Western medicine before going on to specialize in acupuncture. This combined training may require six thousand hours or more. The first standard for formal training leading to licensure/certification in acupuncture in the United States was 1,350 hours in California and roughly the same for the NCCAOM exams. This means that there is up to a fourfold difference of formal training hours for those first generations of licensed/certified acupuncturists compared to those originally trained in the Far East. This difference is at least partly made up today by the amount of experience those trained under lesser hours have obtained. I was trained under the early standard of 1,350 hours required in California at that time, and while I may envy the more extensive formal education of those entering this profession today, I would not trade it for my nearly twenty years of clinical experience.

The variation in formal training among licensed/certified acupuncturists is an understandable aspect of the growing pains of an entirely new (to the Western world) health care field. This is especially true when you consider the great resistance and skepticism that existed within the mainstream medical establishment regarding acupuncture. The acupuncture profession had to fight for every state to allow acupuncture specialists to legally practice there. I am quite proud of the work the acupuncture profession has accomplished in establishing standards for education, schools, and exams. We still have some work to do, especially in regard to working out differences between California and the other states that license/certify acupuncturists and getting those last ten states to formally recognize acupuncture specialists. But the standards established and steadily raised over the last thirty years have done an admirable job in assuring that Americans have access to competently trained acupuncture specialists.

REGULATIONS FOR MEDICAL DOCTORS AND OSTEOPATHS PRACTICING ACUPUNCTURE

As mentioned earlier, the vast majority of states allow medical doctors and osteopaths to practice acupuncture, most without requiring any formal training or examination. One state (Hawaii) does not allow M.D.s or D.O.s to practice acupuncture unless they have obtained a valid license as an acupuncture specialist, as described earlier. A few states require some education in the subject, and fewer still require some sort of examination to be passed. The primary organization for M.D.s and D.O.s who practice acupuncture is the American Academy of Medical Acupuncture (AAMA). In their position paper, this group bills itself as the "sole physician-only acupuncture organization in North America," meaning the only acupuncture organization whose members are limited to medical doctors and osteopaths. This group takes pains to label what their members do as "medical acupuncture," as opposed to acupuncture done by nonphysician acupuncturists. Their position paper identifies medical acupuncture as "the clinical discipline of acupuncture as practiced by a physician who is also trained and licensed in Western biomedicine." This term has proven popular, as many medical doctors throughout the world who practice acupuncture tend to label their services "medical acupuncture," the exception being those medical doctors in the Far East who are also trained in acupuncture.

The AAMA has two broad categories of members: practice and nonpractice members. Nonpractice members are those who have not yet completed minimum training in medical acupuncture or who have indicated they are not currently practicing medical acupuncture. There are three levels of practice members. *Associate members* have either at least two hundred hours of formal training or two years of experience. *Full members* have at least 220 hours of formal training (120 didactic and 100 clinical) and two years of experience practicing medical acupuncture. Fellows—the highest level—are ABMA certified (see hereafter) and have five years of Western medical practice experience, including two or more years practicing medical acupuncture, or are board certified in their specialty, and (1) have at least four years of clinical experience in medical acupuncture after graduation from a medical acupuncture course or (2) have published or had accepted for publication an acupuncture-related article in a recognized medical periodical or (3) have at least ten hours of experience teaching medical professionals on acupuncture-related topics. The AAMA practice members are listed on their referral database, while affiliate, international affiliate, and student members are not. At this writing, the AAMA's total membership is at over 1,800, with approximately 1,500 practice members.

In the year 2000, the AAMA created the American Board of Medical Acupuncture (ABMA) as an independent entity within the AAMA's corporate structure for the purpose of establishing an examination and certification process for physician (medical) acupuncturists. To become certified by the ABMA, candidates must have medical licenses in good standing and at least three hundred hours of approved acupuncture training—two hundred didactic and one hundred clinical—and then pass an examination administered by the ABMA. Upon completion of these requirements, certification as a diplomate of the American Board of Medical Acupuncture (DABMA) is granted. At the time of this writing, the ABMA lists just over 320 certified (DABMA) physicians and the AAMA just over fifty fellows.

While the AAMA is a private membership organization, and no states require AAMA membership or ABMA certification as a requirement for M.D.s or D.O.s to practice acupuncture, their memberships/certifications offer a degree of assurance that the doctors recognized under this process have undergone some standard of minimum training. These minimum standards were designed to meet or exceed those established by the WHO for medical doctors practicing acupuncture. The WHO actually established two categories of training for physicians utilizing acupuncture; "limited" and "full." The AAMA's minimum requirement of two hundred hours of training meets the hours recommended by the WHO for limited training for physicians. The WHO's recommended full training for physicians practicing acupuncture is a minimum of 1,500 hours—including at least 1,000 hours of practical and clinical training. To the best of my knowledge, no program currently in the United States teaches the WHO's full training for physicians. The WHO recommends that those physicians who take either the limited or full training also pass official examinations.

REGULATIONS FOR CHIROPRACTORS PRACTICING ACUPUNCTURE

In a manner similar to how many states allow medical doctors and osteopaths to practice acupuncture, several states allow chiropractors to practice acupuncture with either no required training or a minimum of anywhere from fifty to two hundred hours. Some chiropractic colleges offer postgraduate certification courses in acupuncture. One school, the Southern California University of the Health Sciences, teaches both an accredited chiropractic and acupuncture program. Those who take the combined training can become licensed as both a chiropractor and a California state and nationally certified acupuncturist. Another resource for chiropractors interested in acupuncture is an organization known as the International Academy of Medical Acupuncture (IAMA). Like the AAMA, the IAMA describes "medical acupuncture" as acupuncture practiced by "physicians," but unlike the AAMA, the IAMA recognizes licensed chiropractors, naturopaths, dentists, and podiatrists as "physicians." So while the AAMA's membership is limited to medical doctors and osteopaths, the IAMA also recognizes those other health care specialties.

The IAMA was originally founded in 1973 as the Academy of Clinical Acupuncture by a chiropractor and (later) NCCAOM-certified acupuncturist named John Amaro, who still runs the Academy. The main purpose of the IAMA is to train health care professionals in various acupuncture techniques. The IAMA also offers fellowships (FIAMA) and diplomate status (Dip.Ac. IAMA). Fellowships are awarded to physicians who complete seven 15-hour didactic modules and 200 hours of documented clinical experience within a one-year period and then pass a competency exam and another exam on clean needle protocols. Diplomates are fellows who submit thirty case history presentations. The IAMA also awards a "certified technician" training to "health care support personnel" such as nurses or physician's assistants, who complete the fellowship didactic program and pass the competency exam.

As is the case for the AAMA memberships or ABMA certifications, no state requires IAMA diplomate or fellowship certification, but this process does signify a degree of training and examination beyond most state requirements for chiropractors. It is also my understanding that some state chiropractic boards have recently begun to offer acupuncture modules. Chiropractors who pass this examination may then be recognized as "board certified in acupuncture," but this certification will not be the same as that of licensed/certified acupuncturists who are board certified by their respective acupuncture boards as acupuncture boards require more extensive training and testing.

REGULATIONS FOR NATUROPATHS PRACTICING ACUPUNCTURE

Approximately a dozen states regulate the practice of naturopathy, and a limited number of these allow naturopaths to practice acupuncture. In the state of Arizona, naturopaths must take an acupuncture exam module as part of their national licensing examination. As far as I was able to determine in my research, no states require any specific hours of training in acupuncture; states leave this training up to the naturopathy schools to decide.

■ REGULATIONS FOR OTHER HEALTH CARE ■ PROFESSIONALS PRACTICING ACUPUNCTURE

In addition to those already mentioned, various other health care professionals are allowed by some states to legally practice acupuncture, although most of these only allow this in some restricted manner. A handful of states allow dentists and podiatrists to practice acupuncture, although most will restrict this practice to dental disorders for dentists and problems of the foot and/or lower leg for podiatrists. Most of those states do not require these doctors to undergo any specified training or examination. A few states allow nurses or physician assistants to practice acupuncture under physician supervision. A couple of states even allow nurses and physician assistants to practice without any required training under the supervision of a physician who is also not required to undergo any formal training—yet these states do not allow licensed/certified acupuncturists to practice!

There are also some states that allow people working in drug treatment programs, usually called drug detox specialists, to perform acupuncture for the sole purpose of helping the treatment of chemical dependency. These specialists are trained in a protocol for treating chemical dependency developed by an organization known as the National Acupuncture Detoxification Association (NADA). The NADA protocol involves using three to five specific acupuncture points found within the cartilage of a person's ears. This is known as auricular (ear) acupuncture. When used in combination with appropriate counseling and support services, the NADA ear-points protocol has proven remarkably effective in improving success rates in a wide range of different chemical dependencies.

▣ RISKS ASSOCIATED WITH ACUPUNCTURE ▣

I have made several statements regarding the relative safety of reaction medicine, including acupuncture. However, no healing method that has the ability to positively change an illness can do so with zero risk. When compared to other healing methods, especially those with better success in treating health problems, acupuncture is remarkably low risk. A recent study published in the January/February 2004 issue of the journal *Alternative Therapies* looked at all reports of adverse events associated with acupuncture in all English-language sources over the last thirty-five years. They found only 202 reported events, which averages out to only six cases per year, throughout twenty-two countries! Most of these reports (124) took place during the ten-year span from 1975 to 1985 when acupuncture first exploded on the scene in the West and training standards were few. Reports of such events have been on the decline, with only fifteen cases being reported in the years 1996–1999.

The risks associated with acupuncture can be divided into two categories: minor and major. Both of those categories were counted in the aforementioned study. Minor risks include such things as bruising, dizziness or fainting, and skin irritation. Major risks include such serious problems as transmitting hepatitis or puncturing internal organs. The minor risks of bruising, dizziness, fainting, and so forth are sometimes unavoidable but quickly resolve with no lasting effects. The major risks involving infection or puncturing sensitive tissues are almost always avoidable and mostly take place because of poor training in acceptable technique, mistakes, or accidents. In other words, when acupuncture is performed the way it is taught in legitimate training programs, major risks are almost zero.

All the known cases of transmitting an infectious disease like hepatitis were found to have occurred when accepted protocols for hygienic use of acupuncture needles were not followed. This risk is now essentially zero with acupuncturists who exclusively use disposable needles, as most of them do. The other type of infection possible with acupuncture is from bacterial infections that can take place from the skin being broken, just as a cut can get infected. The most common form of this—although it is nonetheless extremely rare—can happen with certain techniques in which a type of tiny needle is left within the body for days at a time. One of these techniques involves leaving very small pins in the ears covered with tape. Another type, popular in Japan or among those utilizing Japanese-style techniques, uses tiny needles that are slid just under the skin on regular body points. Because these devices are left under the skin for extended periods of time, they have a greater risk of becoming infected. Care should be taken to keep the sites of these needles clean, including making sure your hands are clean if instructed to stimulate (press) these points from time to time. There should also be clear instructions for removing these devices, as some of the body-type (Japanese) devices have been found to become lodged beneath the skin if forgotten and not removed.

The very rare but serious risk of puncturing sensitive tissues usually involves needling deeper than accepted standards. The proper depth of needle insertion is an important aspect of all well-trained acupuncturists' education. While there have been instances of acupuncture causing a puncture in an internal organ, or to the spinal cord or a major vessel, such incidents occur far less often than one in several million acupuncture treatments. Research also suggests this already rare complication is less likely to occur now that minimum standards of formal training programs for acupuncture have been increased. Puncturing a lung can lead to pneumothorax or collapsed lung. It should be noted, however, that the vast majority of cases of pneumothorax do not involve acupuncture, and some happen for no known reason, so it is possible that an acupuncture patient who suffers a collapsed lung may have developed it for other reasons.

While almost all major risks are avoidable by the practitioner ob-

THE HEALING POWER OF ACUPRESSURE AND ACUPUNCTURE

taining and following accepted training, in extremely rare instances complications could occur despite following established protocols. Some people could have major blood vessels in areas where they are not normally found or other sorts of physical abnormalities that could lead to freak accidents. The odds of this happening are infinitesimal but not impossible. Other factors to consider are the use of blood-thinning medications or pacemakers. Patients should inform their acupuncturists of either of these. In the case of blood-thinning medication, the acupuncturist should avoid bleeding techniques. If a patient has a pacemaker, electrical acupuncture should not be used, especially around the chest area.

While acupuncture can cause pain during the treatment, it very rarely causes any residual pain, as often happens, for example, after getting a shot. If the area where acupuncture was applied stays painful long after a needle is removed, this is a sign of injury to the local tissues. Let your acupuncturist know if this happens, as he or she may be able to instruct you on how to speed recovery from this. Most pain involved with acupuncture, including the very rare injuries just described, can be greatly reduced with the use of thinner needles. There is a wide range of needle sizes, including thickness. Many acupuncturists today prefer to use thinner needles, although some prefer the thicker ones. If you find acupuncture uncomfortable, discuss this with your acupuncturist. If you are not satisfied with what you are told, look for another acupuncturist who uses thinner needles. The thinner needles favored by many acupuncturists (and their patients) can be as thin as a human hair!

The bottom line on the risks involved with acupuncture, then, is that while minor, temporary complications such as bruising or dizziness following treatment are sometimes unavoidable, the more serious and extremely rare risks can mostly be avoided by the use of disposable needles and the adequate training in proper needling technique that comes with higher standards of training.

▣ How to Find a Qualified Acupressurist ▣

There are no states that require any sort of licensing or certification for one to practice acupressure. Some states or counties consider acupressure to be an aspect of massage therapy and require a massage therapy license for those practicing acupressure. Many massage schools teach courses in acupressure as part of their overall massage training, but such courses are not standardized or approved by any outside accrediting agency (that I know of). Thus, as in the case of acupuncture, there is a wide variation in training, experience, and skill among those who practice acupressure.

As mentioned in chapter 3, most acupuncturists practice some amount of acupressure, although few have extensive training in that practice. If you are seeking acupressure from an acupuncturist, ask how many acupressure treatments the practitioner averages in a day or a week. Some may only do one a month or less and only then on a patient who is not willing to be treated with acupuncture. Other acupuncturists may have made acupressure an integral part of their practice and have a good amount of experience with it. While all acupuncturists should have a reasonable level of basic skill in acupressure, those with the most training and experience are likely to do a better job of it, just as those acupuncturists with the most training and experience usually do a better job with that therapy.

Many massage therapists also offer acupressure services and have had some training in it during their schooling although, as mentioned earlier, the level of this training can vary greatly. As most massage therapists need to develop sensitive hands, they are well suited to learn acupressure techniques, although they also need to learn a good amount of Chinese medicine theory to become truly proficient. Again, ask about how much training the practitioner has had in acupressure and how many acupressure sessions he or she performs on average.

There is one organization that specializes in acupressure and Asian bodywork therapies and certifies their members in that specialty: the American Organization for Bodywork Therapies of Asia (AOBTA). The AOBTA has members known as certified practitioners, who must demonstrate at least five hundred hours of training from an AOBTA-approved program, and associate members, with at least 150 hours of training from approved courses. In addition to AOBTA, the NCCAOM, the organization that certifies diplomates in acupuncture, also certifies diplomates in Asian bodywork therapy, designated by the title Dipl.ABT (NCCAOM). NCCAOM diplomates in Asian bodywork therapy must complete five hundred hours of approved training and pass a written examination administered by the NCCAOM. Both AOBTA and NCCAOM will refer prospective patients to their certified practitioners/diplomates. Because not all NCCAOM ABT diplomates will choose to join the AOBTA and AOBTA certified practitioners are not limited to NCCAOM ABT diplomates, you may want to check with both organizations to get the most comprehensive list of qualified practitioners. While no states require a license to practice acupressure alone, about nine states require NCCAOM certification in Asian bodywork therapy to practice acupressure as a form of Asian bodywork.

■ RISKS ASSOCIATED WITH ACUPRESSURE ■

The major risks involved with acupressure are even lower than those associated with acupuncture. As with acupuncture, most of these risks can be avoided with proper training. As with acupuncture, minor risks involve such things as bruising and dizziness. Some acupressure treatment techniques are rather painful—others are not. More serious risks can occur if too forceful a pressure is applied to the spine or ribs, especially if the patient has osteoporosis (brittle bones). Forceful pressure should be used with caution over the abdomen, breasts, and orifices, and avoided at areas involving sprains, swellings, lymph glands, broken skin or skin disorders, tumors, or fractures.

▪ HOW TO FIND A QUALIFIED PRACTITIONER ▪ OF CHINESE HERBAL REMEDIES

As with acupressure, most states do not require any sort of licensing or certification for the practice of prescribing Chinese herbal remedies. Several of the states that license/certify acupuncture specialists include the use of Chinese herbs in those specialists' scope of practice. In my state, California, for example, licensed acupuncturists are trained in the use of Chinese herbs under education guidelines set forth by the state, and the subject of the correct use of Chinese herbs is an integral part of the state licensing examinations. Some of the states that require passing NCCAOM acupuncture examinations also allow acupuncture specialists to utilize Chinese herbs. In addition to administering examinations for acupuncture and Asian bodywork therapies, the NCCAOM also administers an examination for Chinese herbologist. Most of the states that include Chinese herbs in an acupuncturist's scope of practice require these acupuncturists to have passed the NCCAOM's Chinese herbology examination.

▪ RISKS ASSOCIATED WITH CHINESE HERBS ▪

Over literally thousands of years of use, the Chinese and other peoples of the Far East have developed the largest and most comprehensive body of knowledge on natural substances for medicinal use the world has ever known. In addition to learning how to get the most benefit from these natural remedies, they have also learned a great deal about how to use them in a safe manner.

The Chinese divided many of the more than 10,000 substances they identified for medicinal use into three categories they called superior, middle, and inferior. These classifications were a sort of combination of the sentiment expressed by two sayings we know in the West: "An ounce of prevention is worth a pound of cure" and "First, do no harm." The superior herbs were those that were primarily used for prevention by helping to brace up or "tonify" one's health before one got too ill. These herbs were also the safest, and many very close in nature to foods. These substances qualify as reaction medicines. The inferior herbs were those that were the most powerful in their ability to change the course of an established disease. Some of these substances qualify as action medicines similar to modern drugs and carry the highest risk of undesirable side effects. These are the types of substances modern drug companies would be interested in as potential sources of new drugs. The middle herbs were those in the middle between these two—substances that had some potential for undesirable side effects but not as serious as inferior herbs and able to treat illness but not as powerfully as inferior herbs. Some of these herbs are reaction medicines, others action medicines.

The classification of these medicinal substances into these categories shows how much emphasis the Chinese placed on both prevention and safety. Because of this emphasis, they not only did a very good job of learning which substances posed what degree of risk but also learned how to work with the level of risk, by developing both protocols for dosages and ways to process and combine herbs to reduce their negative effects while maintaining their medicinal effects. However, understanding these risks takes training. I mentioned in the last chapter that most Chinese herbs consumed in the United States are taken without advice from a professional trained in their use. As is the case with acupuncture and acupressure, most of the risk associated with Chinese herbs can be greatly reduced if they are taken as directed by a trained professional.

The minor risks associated with Chinese herbs center mostly around symptoms of the digestive system—upset stomach, diarrhea or constipation, and so on. These problems are similar to the consequences of eating foods that "don't agree with you" and usually subside quickly as your body adjusts to the herbs. These symptoms can happen with herbs from any of the three categories. The major risks associated with Chinese herbs are almost entirely from those classified as inferior herbs. As with modern drugs, some of these substances are toxic to the body and can build up within the system and cause damage to a range of internal organs, especially the kidneys, liver, and brain. These substances especially, should only be taken under the direction of a trained professional, just as prescription drugs should only be taken under the direction of a licensed physician. I want to emphasize however, that the number of substances used in Chinese medicine that carry this level of risk so common in modern drug therapy is only a small fraction of the thousands of substances that make up the whole of Chinese herbals.

Another source of risk associated with Chinese herbs has to do with manufacturers of Chinese herb products that falsely label their products. Some Chinese herbal products have been found to contain Western pharmaceutical drugs. The most dangerous of these have come from fly-by-night companies who sell mostly by mail order, including on the Internet. These are criminals who seek to take advantage of uninformed consumers. Most of these will advertise miraculous cures for specific diseases, such as diabetes, AIDS, or cancer. In contrast, there are many highly reputable Chinese herb companies out there too; these, however, will not claim to be able to cure serious disease. A trained Chinese herbalist will know what companies are reputable and trustworthy and will be able to advise you what to trust and what to avoid.

Another category of false labeling of Chinese herb products is far less dangerous but still a cause for concern. These are products that come from the Far East, including some from China. There are many companies that sell Chinese herbal products that they label "patent" products, although these products are not under legal patents as we use that term in the United States. These products are similar to our "over-the-counter" medicines, remedies that are well known to consumers and are purchased without prescription. A tiny minority of these products have been found to contain some Western pharmaceuticals, although mostly much more mild types such as antihistamines or aspirin. The Chinese government has been cracking down on these companies, and such problems are far less common today. Again, those who are trained and work professionally with these substances will be the best informed about which companies have the best reputations.

Given that the number of substances used in Chinese herbal medicine is so vast, it is impossible to be 100 percent sure that every possible risk has been discovered. It is possible that some risk involved with some of these substances has not yet been clearly understood over the generations of their use within Chinese medicine. The same is true however, for the drugs that we take every day that have been approved for sale by our government's system of testing and oversight. It is my firm belief, however, that Chinese herbs, in the hands of a professional trained in their use, afford us a healing resource that is far safer on average than our current Western drug remedies. This does not mean, however, that Chinese herbs are always more effective. As powerful action medicine agents, many Western drugs are more effective for serious disorders than even the most powerful Chinese herbs. A trained professional will be able to work with you to know what conditions the safer Chinese remedies are suited for and when the higher-risk drugs are needed.

Finally, there can be concerns about interactions between the use of Chinese herbs and medications, usually referred to as "herb/drug" interactions. Mixing different medications, whether they be herbs with drugs, drugs with other drugs, or herbs with other herbs, will necessarily carry some risk of a combined effect that poses health risks beyond that of the individual medications. Very little hard evidence exists to prove that traditional Chinese herb formulas, taken as directed by a trained professional, will cause adverse herb/drug interactions. This question is actually very difficult to prove scientifically beyond doubt, so most professionals prescribing Chinese herbs err on the side of caution and avoid using herbs that are even *suspected* of having the potential to interact with other drugs. Those trained in the use of Chinese herbs have very good resources available to them to keep current on suspected herb/drug interactions, and this is another reason one should seek the advice of a trained professional before using Chinese herbs for treating health matters. *Always remember to inform your herbalist of medications you are taking, and your medical doctor about herbs you are taking.*

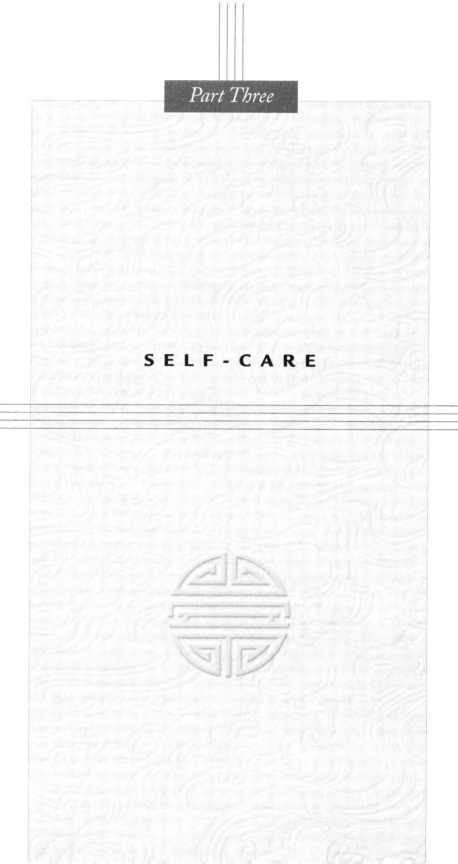

Part Three

SELF-CARE

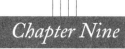

Chapter Nine

TREATING YOURSELF,

FAMILY, AND FRIENDS

WITH ACUPRESSURE

IN THIS CHAPTER, I WILL REVIEW some acupressure points that you can use on yourself or on another to treat some common conditions. This will be a brief review of a handful of the most important points and is not meant to be comprehensive or in any way to replace the services of a health care professional. Some precautions before we start: you should not perform acupressure on broken skin, inflamed tissues such as a sprained joint, directly on lymph glands or other nodules under the skin, or when under the influence of drugs or alcohol, or extremely fatigued. Some acupressure points, most of which are on the lower extremities, should not be stimulated during pregnancy, especially in the late stages, as they might encourage uterine contractions. (Conversely, points on the upper part of the body can help prevent miscarriage.) I will identify the points that should be avoided during pregnancy by marking them "(contraindicated during pregnancy)."*

I often tell acupuncture and acupressure students that learning how to feel for problem spots and then how to stimulate them is just as important as learning the location and indications of classic points. Before we go on to consider the locations and indications of some of these classic points, a few words about the best way to touch problem spots will be helpful.

The most important skill to develop to be successful with any system of touch therapy, including acupressure, is to be able to feel what the flesh you are touching is trying to tell you. Nature endowed our bodies with a strong inclination to stay healthy, so when we touch problems spots in the flesh, these spots will try to tell us what to do with them. This type of feedback is somewhat similar to what can be experienced in sensual touch—the flesh will tell you what it desires if you are tuned in. Let me stress, however, that this analogy to sensual touch is only an analogy; the type of touch helpful for healing is very different from that helpful for sexual gratification. Healing touch often unlocks deep-seated energy blockages that connect across the spectrum of body/mind/spirit. There is nothing titillating about this type of touch. If applying touch therapy causes any sexual arousal in either the patient or the therapist, the touch is on the wrong wavelength and is not therapeutic.

In order to develop the ability to feel what the flesh is trying to tell you, you need to be patient. You may not be able to feel any feedback at first, but if you just relax, breathe evenly, keep a moderate pressure on the point, and hold it there, the feedback will usually come. It is always

*The precaution regarding some points being contraindicated during pregnancy is a good example of the zero tolerance toward side effects typical in acupuncture/acupressure. While it is possible that some of these points could cause a pregnant woman to begin uterine contractions, this could only happen in very rare instances. Acupressure and especially acupuncture are sometimes used to help facilitate delivery, but even when one is trying to make this reaction happen in a patient ready to deliver, it will not always cause this to happen.

better to apply too little pressure than too much, so another important principle to follow is to slowly increase the amount of pressure up to the level at which the point starts to feel slightly uncomfortable. As an example of what I mean by this, let's consider how to find and apply pressure to four points that will then help you be able to find the other points we will consider. Start with feeling these points on yourself before you try them on anyone else. This will give you an idea of what it feels like to have these points stimulated and so help you to get a sense of the feedback you should feel when you apply these points to another. Let's start with what is perhaps the most famous of all acupuncture/acupressure points.

Virtually every book on acupressure will prominently list the point located between the thumb and index finger known as Large Intestine 4 (contraindicated during pregnancy); it is a point well known for its use in treating headaches and tooth and facial pain. This point lies directly over a large nerve and is thus quite sensitive when pressed or needled. In order to find this point, rest your thumb and index finger together, creating a crease between the two. Large Intestine 4 is at the end of the crease. Stimulate this point by placing the tip of your thumb at the end of this crease and the tip of your index finger underneath this point. Gently pinch between the two (see the illustration below) and then gradually increase the pressure. Given that this point is so sensitive, you will feel a strong sensation with even light to moderate pressure.

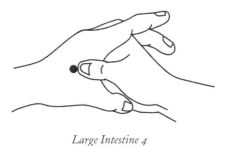

Large Intestine 4

Practice slightly shifting your pressure, trying to find the bull's-eye—the exact spot that is the most sensitive. Once you find this most sensitive spot, use as little pressure as possible to make it feel *slightly* uncomfortable and hold it there for thirty seconds. Remember, it is always best to use too little pressure rather than too much.

After finding and stimulating this spot for thirty seconds, rest for another thirty seconds and then repeat a second time. Now repcat this on your other hand. By the time you finish stimulating both hands in this manner, you should feel a somewhat odd feeling—a little light-headed or almost like being lightly drugged. Because reactions vary so much with each individual, this feeling will vary somewhat from person to person, but most people will find they feel a little strange after stimulating these points.

Most of the other points we will learn to use will not be as sensitive and easy to find as Large Intestine 4 but should give a lesser version of the same features of that point. They should all have a bulls'-eye spot that is more sensitive than the area immediately around it, and most will cause a reaction that leaves you feeling relaxed or a little light-headed. Now let's find another point that is less sensitive than the first but offers a good example of how some acupressure points can feel as though they are custom-made for one's fingertip.

This next point is known as Liver 3 (contraindicated for pregnancy), and its location is very similar to Large Intestine 4, except it is at the base of the big and second toes instead of the thumb and index finger. Find this point by pressing your fingertip at the webbing between the big and second toe and then slide it upward toward your ankle. You will feel the spacing between those two bones narrow as they start to come closer together like a V. Liver 3 is located in the last bit of soft flesh before the bones come together.

In addition to being useful for pain in the feet, this point helps to reduce stress, lower blood pressure, in general lowering excess energy

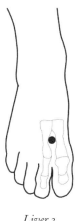

Liver 3

in the head that may cause headaches or eye problems. It also treats menstrual problems and problems of the external genitalia and hernia. Press this point with the tip of your thumb, using gradually increasing pressure with both hands to stimulate both feet if you wish. While not as sensitive as Large Intestine 4, this point is somewhat sensitive, and you should feel some discomfort with moderate pressure. Again, shift your pressure while feeling for the bull's-eye and then use as little pressure as possible to maintain a slight discomfort. Hold for thirty to sixty seconds and then wait thirty seconds before repeating. If you only did one foot, repeat the procedure on the other. You should again feel relaxed or even a little light-headed afterward.

LARGE INTESTINE 4 *(contraindicated during pregnancy)*
Location: In the webbing between the thumb and index finger, at the end of the crease made when those two are pressed together.
Technique: Squeeze between the thumb and index finger with light to moderate pressure; hold for thirty seconds. Repeat two additional times.
Used for: Thumb pain, headache, dental and facial pain, general pain relief.

LIVER 3 *(contraindicated during pregnancy)*

Location: In the depression just past the union of the first and second metatarsal bones.

Technique: Press downward with thumb or fingertip with moderate pressure for thirty to sixty seconds. Repeat two additional times.

Used for: Foot pain, headache, red eyes, irritability, insomnia, menstrual problems, pain or other problems of the external genitalia, hernia, some digestive disorders.

The first of our next two points, similar to Liver 3, is also found in a V-shaped depression, except this one is in a much smaller depression between two tendons. Known as Lung 7, this point is located just above the base of the thumb on the side of the wrist and can be found with a simple trick: join the webbing between the thumb and index finger of your two hands so that the index finger of one hand rests on the bone by the wrist of the other, pointing toward the elbow. Where the tip of your index finger rests will be a small depression on the bone between two small tendons on either side of your fingertip. Don't try to reach up your forearm when you do this; just let the tip of your index finger lightly rest on the bone (see the illustration below).

It may take a little probing before you find this depression. Once you find it, press in, either with the tip of your index finger or the tip of you thumb. Try to relax the hand you are pressing against. This

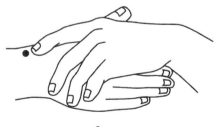

Lung 7

point will not be as sensitive and easy to find as Large Intestine 4 or
Liver 3, but if you find the depression, just press around the middle of
it looking for the bulls'-eye, and you should find a slightly sensitive
spot. Hold pressure there for thirty to sixty seconds, release, and repeat
after a 30-second rest, as you did earlier, and repeat for the other hand.
While the reaction you get from this point will usually not be as strong
as our first two points, you should again feel as though something has
affected you more than you would expect from just pressing a point by
the wrist. This point is used for local wrist or thumb pain as well as the
beginning stages of respiratory problems and certain headaches and
neck pains. As Lung 7 is a little tricky to find, if you can find and get a
reaction out of it, you should be able to find and stimulate most of the
other points we will consider.

The last of our first set of points can also be very sensitive, especially for women. This point is called Spleen 6 (contraindicated for
pregnancy) and is considered to be a point where the three yin qi pathways of the leg meet, and so stimulating this point can have a balancing effect on these three pathways. All of these pathways are closely
connected with the sexual organs and the reproductive essence and
thus can be helpful in balancing hormones. As women tend to be quite
susceptible to hormone imbalances, Spleen 6 will be more sensitive for
most women than men on average, although many men will find this
a sensitive spot also. Learning how to find this point will help one to
find many other points because it is found by using a very helpful system that is used to measure the distance between body landmarks and
points or between different points.

Although simple aids to finding points like those we used for
Large Intestine 4 and Lung 7 are very helpful, not every point has similar simple methods to help us find them. The Chinese developed an
ingenious measuring method to designate the location of all the
acupuncture/acupressure points, based on dividing the different por-
tions of the body into equal divisions called body inches, as well as a

convenient shortcut for measuring body inches using the fingers (see the illustration below).

To find Spleen 6, we want to find the spot three body inches above the big bone on the inside of the ankle (medial malleoulus) just at the border of the shin bone (tibia). To do this, we take four fingers and rest the little finger on the tip of the ankle bone. The spot where the index finger touches is approximately three body inches above the ankle bone (see the illustration on page 165).

Spleen 6 is right at the border of where the shin bone meets the

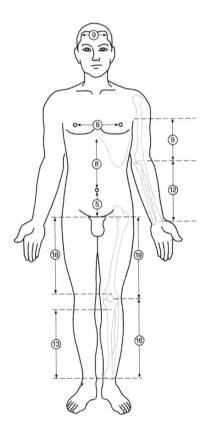

Various body inches

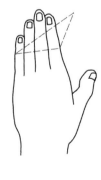

Quick measurement to approximate 3 body inches

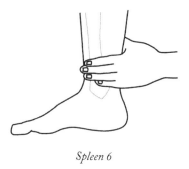

Spleen 6

muscle around it. Press in with your thumb, being very gentle, as you may find it surprisingly sore. Don't press longer than thirty seconds the first time you press this point, then let it rest for thirty to sixty seconds before pressing again. The second time you press this spot it may be quite tender and require less pressure. Once you have stimulated Spleen 6 a few times over several days, it will probably become less sensitive (a good sign) and you can then press it for longer periods of time.

LUNG 7

Location: In the depression between two tendons on the bone two finger widths (1½ body inches) above the base of the thumb, found by joining webbing of index finger and thumbs together, under the tip of the index finger.

Technique: Press inward with moderate pressure for 30 seconds. Repeat two additional times.

Used for: Wrist and thumb pain; beginning of cold or flu; respiratory problems; headache, especially with neck pain.

SPLEEN 6 *(contraindicated during pregnancy)*

Location: Four finger widths (three body inches) above the tip of the inner ankle bone, where the flesh meets the edge of the shin bone (tibia).

Technique: Press inward with light, gradual pressure for 30 seconds. Be careful, as this point may be very tender. Repeat two additional times.

Used for: Local lower leg problems, many female hormone problems, speeding labor (child delivery), building energy, digestive disorders, diabetes, many urologic and genital problems.

I chose to start with these four points because they represent a pretty good cross-section of the range of different characteristics of acupuncture/acupressure points; both in the sensations they usually cause and in the methods used to locate them. I also chose them because they represent a nice mixture of points on both the upper and lower extremities. The goal of every therapy in Chinese medicine is to balance yin and yang by adding to that which has too little and taking away from that which has too much. While acupressure is a very safe procedure, it does effect a person's qi, so if someone is experiencing an imbalance of too little qi in the head, for example, and points on the lower extremities are stimulated, this may further draw qi from the head toward the lower part of the body. A good rule to remember then, unless you are certain you understand the imbalance, is to stimulate both upper and lower points to avoid moving too much energy in the wrong direction.

The first two points, Large Intestine 4 and Liver 3, are often used in combination with each other to balance the lower with the upper (yin with yang) and are known as the Four Gates. Just doing acupressure on these points regularly can help treat a range of problems and help prevent even more. Adding the next two points, Lung 7 and Spleen 6, really make for a good tuneup. In the next section, I will list several additional points and their locations and indications. The skills you have begun to learn with finding the first four points should make the rest go more easily.

Our next two points, Bladder 2 and Stomach 2, are good points for both eye and sinus disorders as well as certain headaches. While you can stimulate these points in any position, a good method when pressing these on yourself is to place your elbows on a tabletop, with the tips of your thumbs pointing upward. Tilt your head forward so your thumb tips rest in the points (two at a time, of course) and let gravity lower your head onto your thumbs to find the right pressure (see the illustrations). If you have sinus problems, add Lung 7 to these points. For treating eye problems, add Liver 3.

BLADDER 2

Location: At the inner border of the eyebrow in a small depression next to a ridge of bone (supraobital notch).

Technique: Press inward with a moderate pressure for 30–60 seconds. Repeat two times.

Used for: Eye and sinus problems, including sinus headaches.

STOMACH 2

Location: About one finger-width below lower border of the eye, directly below the pupil, in a hollow in the center of the cheekbone.

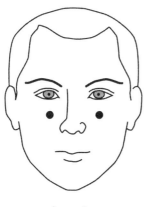

Stomach 2

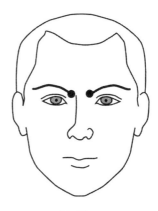

Bladder 2

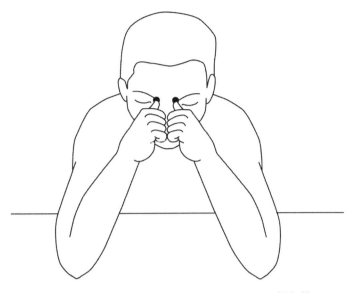

Using thumbs with aid of gravity to press Stomach 2 and Bladder 2

Technique: Press inward with moderate pressure for 30–60 seconds. Repeat two times.

Used for: Another good point for sinus and eye problems.

Let's move on to the next two points, Triple Heater 5 and Pericardium 6. These points are located at the same position just above the wrist, one on the underside, the other on the top side. Both of these points are located on the midline two body inches above the wrist crease, which can be found by placing the index, middle, and ring fingers on the crease (see the illustrations). Both can be used for treating wrist, hand, and forearm (local) problems, as well as a host of conditions in different areas of the body. Triple Heater 5 can be used at the beginning of a cold or flu and for headaches, especially those with neck pain. Pericardium 6 is useful for problems in the chest region, including asthma and angina and feelings of chest tightness. This point also

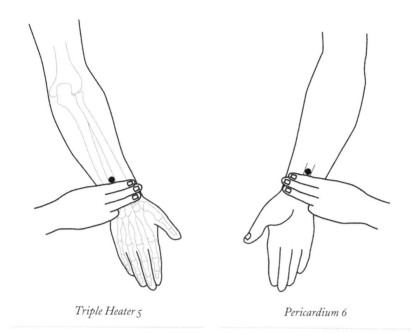

Triple Heater 5   *Pericardium 6*

helps calm the mind and can help insomnia. It is best known for its re-markable effectiveness in treating nausea. This is the spot that the popular types of seasickness wristbands stimulate. When used to-gether, Pericardium 6 and Triple Heater 5 help to balance the yin and yang of the body, especially the upper body.

TRIPLE HEATER 5

Location: Three finger widths up from the wrist crease in the center of the top side of the forearm, between the two bones (radius and ulna).

Technique: Press straight downward with the tip of you thumb with moderate pressure for thirty to sixty seconds. Repeat two times. This point can be used together with Pericardium 6 by pinching the two points between the tip of the middle and index finger.

Used for: Hand, wrist, and forearm pains, first stages of colds and flu, headaches with neck pain.

PERICARDIUM 6

Location: Three finger widths up from the wrist crease on the underside of the forearm, between the two tendons that run down the
center of the arm just above the wrist.

Technique: Press inward with the tip of the thumb with moderate to
strong pressure.

Used for: Hand, wrist, and forearm pains, nausea, chest tightness,
asthma, insomnia.

The next two points we will consider are located in the chest region and can help problems associated with the lungs and heart. If you
remember the correspondences of the five-phase table in chapter 4, the
autumn/metal/lung correspondence is also associated with the sinus,
large intestine, and the skin, so our first chest point, Lung 1, can be
useful for those problems also. This point is located just outside the
space between the first and second rib, which is about an inch below
the middle of the collarbone (clavicle). The next point, Conception
Vessel 17, is located in the center of the breastbone (sternum) on a line
level with the nipples or the space between the fourth and fifth ribs
(see the illustration). This point is also used for lung problems but can
be helpful for heart conditions as well. As the heart is associated with
the mental realm, this point can also help emotional problems. This is
an especially important point for females, not only for breast problems, including breast milk problems for breast-feeding mothers, but
also for overall hormone balance.

LUNG 1

Location: Three finger widths (two body inches) lateral to the nipple,
one inch below the clavicle, just lateral to the first and second rib.

Technique: Probe around this spot with light pressure. You should find
a slight knot in the muscle (pectoral). Press this spot inward,

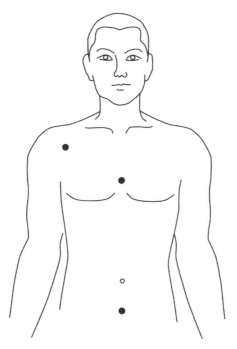

Lung 1 (below collarbone)
Conception Vessel 17 (center of breastbone)
Conception Vessel 4 (below navel)

toward the chest, with gradual pressure until slightly sore. Hold for thirty to sixty seconds. Repeat two more times.

Used for: Lung problems, including cough, asthma, skin problems, and constipation and/or diarrhea.

Conception Vessel 17

Location: In the center of the breastbone (sternum), level with the space between the fourth and fifth rib, which is on line with the nipples (except for women with developed breast).

Technique: Press downward with thumb with light to moderate pressure. Do not press too hard, as this can hurt the tissue here, leaving it quite sore. Press for thirty seconds; repeat two times. After pressing, rub this area lightly to help smooth over any soreness.

Used for: Heart, lung, and emotional problems, breast pain and fibroids, lactation problems, women's hormone problems.

Our last two points can also be used for a host of problems but are especially important spots for helping to build energy levels in the body. The first of these, Conception Vessel 4, aids the body's production of energy, while the second, Stomach 36, mainly helps the circulation of the energy already produced.

CONCEPTION VESSEL 4 *(contraindicated during pregnancy)*
Location: On the centerline of the lower abdomen, four finger widths (three body inches) below the navel.

Technique: This point is best pressed while lying on your back with your knees slightly elevated to relax the abdominal muscles. Press with light to moderate pressure downward for thirty seconds, then release gradually. Repeat two times, then rub this area in a circular motion with the palm of your hand for thirty seconds.

Used for: Many types of reproductive, urinary, and digestive problems, low back pain; especially known for treating early morning diarrhea and helping produce energy.

STOMACH 36 *(contraindicated during pregnancy)*
Location: Four finger widths (three body inches) below the lower edge of the kneecap, and one finger width lateral to the shinbone between the two bones of the lower leg (see the illustration).

Technique: Press with moderate to strong pressure inward with your thumb and hold for thirty seconds. Repeat two times. You may feel a sensation radiating toward your toes.

Used for: A famous point for increasing energy, especially circulation for tired legs and feet, this point is also used for stomach or other digestive disorders, leg problems, and general pain relief.

The one dozen points we have reviewed represent barely one-thirtieth of the classic "primary" acupuncture/acupressure points and so we have only touched the surface of what can be done with this system of healing. Despite this, by using different combinations of these twelve points, it is possible to help a pretty wide range of problems. Each point has the potential to help problems associated with the area surrounding the point itself (called "local" treatment) and a range of problems associated with each point by virtue of holistic interconnected relationships (sometimes referred to as "distal" treatment). Some points, such as Bladder 2 and Stomach 2, are mostly used as local treatments, for facial, sinus, and eye problems, and not so much for treating interconnected things such as bladder or stomach problems, although they could be used for this. Other points, such as Spleen 6 or Stomach 36, are mostly used for treating internal problems via holistic interconnected influences and not as much for local disorders, although they could be used locally. Learning the details of the relative therapeutic strengths of different points and their endless possible combinations is literally a lifelong endeavor. In the next chapter, I will explain a very useful technique for treating pain of many types, and then I will discuss how to use the twelve points I have been reviewing for treating several common health problems.

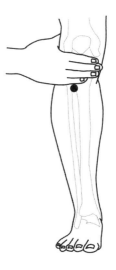

Stomach 36

173

Chapter Ten

TREATING COMMON

HEALTH PROBLEMS

WITH ACUPRESSURE

IN ADDITION TO USING SPECIFIC acupressure points, there are some simple techniques that can be applied to locate helpful points for specific problems, especially for treating pain. The techniques I will explain here all follow yin/yang logic: everything has an opposite partner. When you look at the body (or any three-dimensional object, for that matter), you can apply the yin/yang system of contrasting opposites and label the body as having a left side and a right side, a front and a back, and a top and a bottom. The fourth yin/yang pair, of surface and interior, also exists; in fact, it is why some internal problems cause sore spots on the surface—but we will not use that fourth yin/yang pair for this exercise.

The first yin/yang pairing we will consider is the left with the right. Say, for example, you have a pain in your right knee. The first thing you want to do is to gently but firmly probe the area of pain, trying to find the bull's-eye spot—the one spot that seems to be the epicenter of the pain. (Don't worry if you find more than one such spot; you can apply this same technique to more than a single spot.) Once you locate this spot, note its location, and then try to find the exactly corresponding location on your left (opposite) knee. You should find that the corresponding location on the opposite side of the body will have a spot that is more tender than usual—a hidden sore spot, as described in chapter 3. You can then press this spot with your thumb or fingertip, as I described in the previous chapter. Although you should still be careful to not press too hard (remember, it is better to press too gently than to press too firmly), one of the great advantages of using this "opposite-side" form of treatment is that it is less likely that you might overdo it and cause any harm, as can happen if you overdo pressure on the main area of pain.

This left/right method for finding therapeutic spots can also be applied to other areas of the body besides the limbs. If you have a headache causing pain by your right temple, for example, you could press or rub the same area on the opposite temple. If you strained a muscle in your abdomen, causing a pain two inches to the left of your navel, you could press the corresponding spot two inches to the right of your navel. The key to this treatment is to first try to find the exact spot that seems to be the source of the pain and then find its exact partner on the opposite side of the body.

The next yin/yang pairing involves the relationship between the front and back. If you have a pain in your lower back, you should be able to find a corresponding sore spot at the exact same level in your lower abdomen. A common problem many people develop is a pain between the spine and the edge of their shoulder blade. This spot is very difficult to reach on oneself, and even when this spot is rubbed directly, it can be difficult to ease its pain. If you imagine a straight line drawn through the back to the chest—like the path an arrow would take—

you will find this spot to be very sensitive to moderate pressure. Gently rubbing this sensitive spot on the chest will help the pain in the back to improve.

Our final yin/yang pairing involves the relationship between the top and bottom. This pairing is easiest to imagine in relationship to the upper and lower extremities. Both our arms and legs have very similar compositions of bones and joints in that the arms have shoulder, elbow, wrist, and finger joints, while the legs have hip, knee, ankle, and toe joints. Thus, a pain in your right knee may lead to a hidden sore spot in your right elbow that can be rubbed or pressed to help the knee. Likewise, a pain in your thumb may spawn a sore spot on your big toe, while a corresponding sore spot in your shoulder can accompany a pain in your hip, and so forth. In addition to the pairing of the joints of hip/shoulder, knee/elbow, ankle/wrist, and toes/fingers, there also exists a relationship between the spaces between the joints. Thus, a pain in the middle of your shin can spawn a hidden sore spot in the middle of your forearm.

There are also variations of the aforementioned three yin/yang pairs that can be useful. A variation of the left/right pairing is one in which you use the opposite side of the specific part of the body that is painful instead of the same spot on the opposite side of the body. For example, if you had a pain at the inner corner of your right eye, the left/right opposite technique I described above would be to apply pressure to the same spot on the inner corner of your left (opposite) eye. A variation of this would be to press the corresponding spot at the *outer* corner of the *right* (same) eye. A pain on the outside edge of your left foot could be helped by finding a corresponding spot on the inside edge of the same foot.

In the front/back method I described earlier, I only mentioned points on the front and back of the torso. You can also apply this technique to spots on the limbs. For example, in the last chapter I described the points Triple Heater 5 as located three finger widths above the back of the wrist and Pericardium 6 as located three finger widths above the underside of the wrist—in other words, exactly opposite each other. Using the front/back opposite technique, you could stimulate one of these points if you had a pain in the other. A pain in the muscle in the front of your upper arm (biceps) can be accompanied by a therapeutic hidden sore spot in the opposite muscle in the back of the upper arm (triceps).

In the top/bottom example I described earlier, I only spoke of the extremities because it is easier to describe this technique with that example. A somewhat more difficult variation of using this yin/yang pair involves the torso. In chapter 2, I described how the torso can be divided into three sections; from the throat to the diaphragm (upper), the diaphragm to the navel (middle), and the navel to the pubic region (lower). A pain in the middle of the lower region (below the navel) may be treated by finding a corresponding spot in the middle of the upper region (middle of the chest). A pain in the upper section of the middle region can spawn a corresponding spot in the lower section of the middle region.

Finally, there are a number of complex combinations of yin/yang pairings that can be formulated by mixing the aforementioned trio of left/right, front/back, and top/bottom. Let's consider a painful spot on the right knee. Just below the kneecap (patella) is the patellar tendon, the tendon your doctor likes to tap with a little rubber hammer when checking your reflexes. On either side of that tendon is a depression the Chinese call the "eyes" of the knee—each knee having an "inner" and "outer" eye. If you were to have a pain in the inner eye of your right knee, using the variations of the simple yin/yang correspondences we have been considering leads to a remarkable number of possible therapeutic spots you could press. First, let's review the techniques we considered already. Using the left/right technique, you could press the inner eye of the left (opposite) knee or the outer eye of the right (same) knee. Using the front/back technique, you would probe for a tender spot at the same level in the back of the knee. Using the top/ bottom technique involving the limbs, you would look for the corresponding spot by your right elbow just below the "funny bone." Another version of the top/bottom technique would be to find the corresponding spot just above the inner portion of the right kneecap.

Now let's look at some of the combinations we can make out of the foregoing techniques. Around the right knee itself there are a total of eight spots that can be found, including the main pain at the inner knee eye. As discussed earlier, the yin/yang division system leads to quartering. If you were to divide the knee into quarters, with the middle of the kneecap being the middle spot, you end up with upper and lower and left and right quarters. The inner knee eye is in the lower left quarter (as you face the right knee). You can find a useful therapeutic spot at any of the other three quarters—lower right (outer knee eye), upper left, and upper right. Applying the front/back method, you can also quarter the back of the knee and use any of those four spots, giving you eight possible therapeutic spots. Next, you can apply the same model to the left knee, giving you upper and lower and left and right quarters in both the front and back of the knee. This makes 16

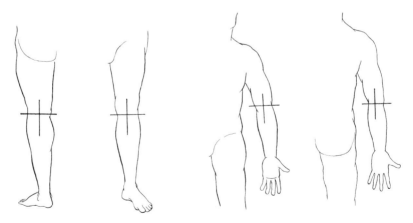

Quartering the front and back of the knee and elbow

possible therapeutic spots. Now apply this system of quartering to the right and left elbows, giving you 16 more points, for a total of thirty-two possible therapeutic spots!

Those with a lot of experience with acupressure and acupuncture who utilize this yin/yang technique will find that, out of these thirty-two possible points, a few usually turn out to be more effective. Using our example of pain in the right inner knee eye, you might find three or four spots that give the best result when stimulated. In addition to stimulating the spot of the main pain, you might find that the same (inner knee eye) spot on the left knee, the spot at the right outer knee eye, the spot directly behind the back of the knee, and the corresponding spot on the right elbow to be the most effective. The amazing thing about the way holistic interconnections work in our bodies is that you can never be sure at any given time just which interconnection will work the best. Some instances of pain in the right inner knee eye might respond best by stimulating the spot at the upper/left/back quadrant of the left elbow, even though that spot is the most removed from the right inner knee eye compared to the rest of the thirty-two. The problem anyone using this system faces, then, is not trying to find any spot that might be useful but rather trying to figure out which of the many possible spots you will choose to use and which ones you won't use. In my experience, the best spots are those that seem to be the most unusually tender—the method, as I suggested in chapter 3, that the ancient Chinese probably used to discover this system of therapy in the first place.

Now let's consider how to use the twelve points we reviewed in the previous chapter for treating a range of different problems. If any health problem you wish to treat involves pain, you can use whichever of these twelve points are indicated for that type of problem and add points from the yin/yang opposite techniques just discussed. For example, in addition to using the points listed hereafter for treating hiatial hernia (which causes pain in the diaphragm region), one could add the opposite point at the same level of the spine (front/back technique) and the spot just above the navel (a variation of the top/bottom technique).

Remember: These recommendations are not a substitute for professional health care but can be used, with the precautions listed in the last chapter, as a supplement to professional care.

Digestive disorders: Hiatial hernia, nausea, stomach/duodenal ulcer, gastritis, colitis, spastic colon, hemorrhoids, diarrhea, and similar digestive disturbances.

Possible points: Stomach 36, Liver 3, Spleen 6, Large Intestine 4, Pericardium 6, Conception Vessel 4.

Explanation of point usage: Both Stomach 36 and Stomach 2 are on the stomach qi pathway that connects internally with the stomach, yet experience has shown Stomach 36 to be especially effective for some stomach problems, while Stomach 2 is not well known for this and so was left off the list of possible points. Liver 3 and Spleen 6 are both used in treating digestive disorders by virtue of the relationship of the spleen/pancreas and liver in the digestive process. Large Intestine 4 is helpful due to its effect on the large intestine and its overall energy-balancing and pain reducing function. Pericardium 6 has been found to be an especially effective point for treating nausea, while Conception Vessel 4 is a good local point for lower abdominal problems.

Respiratory disorders: Asthma, bronchitis, cough, sinus problems including allergic sinusitis and sinus headache, common colds, especially involving upper respiratory infections, pneumonia, and a host of chronic lung disorders.

Possible points: Lung 1, Lung 7, Conception Vessel 17, Pericardium 6, Triple Heater 5, Stomach 2, Bladder 2.

Explanation of point usage: Lung 1 and 7 are on the lung qi pathway and influence the lungs. Conception Vessel 17 is a local point on the breastbone that balances that area. Pericardium 6 is on the pericardium qi pathway and influences the chest, while Triple Heater 5 can be useful in the first stages of a cold or flu. Stomach 2 and Bladder 2 are local points for sinus problems so can be used if the respiratory disorder involves the sinuses.

Headaches: Migraine, tension, cluster, stress, and sinus. Recurring headaches should always be investigated by a trained medical professional. Many migraine headaches involve hormone imbalances, while some headaches may be due to high blood pressure. Other factors can include dietary concerns such as food allergies or sensitivity to caffeine.

Possible points: Stomach 2, Bladder 2, Large Intestine 4, Triple Heater 5, Liver 3, Spleen 6, Conception Vessel 4, Lung 7.

Explanation of point usage: Stomach 2 and Bladder 2 are local points for sinus or frontal headaches. Large Intestine 4 is a powerful pain-relieving point, especially for the head or facial area. Triple Heater 5 is useful for headaches involving neck pain, as the Triple Heater qi pathway runs up the arm to the neck and head. Liver 3 helps attract energy from the head downward and is thus a good point for headaches that involve an excess of energy in the head. Spleen 6 and Conception Vessel 4 both help control hormone imbalances and thus help headaches associated with that problem, especially those around a woman's menstrual cycle. Lung 7 is known as a "command" point for the head and back of the neck, and thus treats problems in those areas.

Reproductive/urogenital disorders: A wide range of disorders involving the reproductive and urinary systems such as infertility, kidney and bladder problems, prostate problems, uterine fibroids, and endometriosis.

Possible points: Conception Vessel 4, Conception Vessel 17, Spleen 6, Liver 3, Large Intestine 4.

Explanation of point usage: Conception Vessel points 4 and 17, by virtue of their connection with Conception Vessel qi pathway, help reproduction problems, especially Conception Vessel 4. Spleen 6 and Liver 3 both are on qi pathways that connect with the reproductive organs, with Spleen 6 being an important hormone-balancing point. Large Intestine 4 can be useful by virtue of being a powerful upper point, hence its ability to help balance the lower with the upper.

MASSAGING THE MERIDIANS

In addition to using specific acupressure points, there are some helpful techniques that can be easily learned that help to encourage the flow of qi within the qi pathways, also known as the "meridians." These massage techniques have been used for centuries in China, especially for daily health maintenance and disease prevention. However, they can also be helpful for treating heath problems, especially when combined with other acupressure or acupuncture techniques, Chinese herbs, and exercise techniques.

In the illustrations, you can see the direction of qi flow within the pathways. The three yang pathways of the hand flow along the outside of the arm toward the head, while three more start in the head area and flow down the torso to the outside of the legs and end at the toes. The three yin pathways of the feet flow up the inside of the leg and end in the chest, while another three start in the chest area and then flow down the inner aspect of the arm and end at the fingers.

A simple massage technique to encourage qi flow is to hold your arm in front of you with your palm facing downward and then, starting at the back of the hand, gently stroke your skin, moving up your

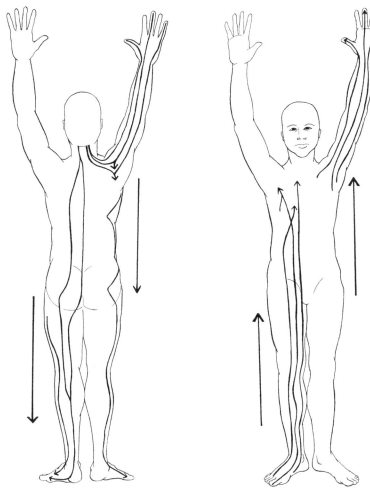

Yang meridians flow from the fingertips to the head and then from the head to the toes.

Yin meridians flow from the toes to the chest and then from the chest to the fingertips.

arm, and continuing until you reach your shoulder. Next, turn your palm facing upward and then stroke down over your inner arm to your palm and fingertips. This should be done as one complete motion, taking just two to three seconds to travel up the arm, turn your hand upward, and then two to three seconds down the arm to the fingertips.

_hen, turn your hand facing downward again and repeat this motion, for a total of twenty times up and down on both arms. The path of your hand stroking up and down your arm should follow the path of the yang and yin meridians shown in the illustration.

The same basic stroking motion can be done with the legs and can be done in either the standing or sitting positions. Start by placing your hand over your big toe and then gently stroke up your inner leg and thigh to your groin area. Then slide your hand over the front of the thigh and out toward your hip and then stroke down your outer leg to the little toe. As with the arms, this upward and downward motion should follow the path seen in the drawings, takes just a few seconds in each direction, and is done in one continuous motion, for a total of 20 times on both legs.

This massage technique is an excellent daily exercise to encourage qi flow, especially if used in combination with some of the twelve points I have discussed. A great five- to ten-minute routine is to do this massage technique, then apply acupressure to the first four points I reviewed in the previous chapter (Large Intestine 4, Liver 3, Lung 7, and Spleen 6), and then repeat the massage technique for a second time.

I hope the foregoing gives you some ideas on how to use acupressure and some insights on how complex this healing system is. While the techniques I described in these last two chapters can prove quite helpful, such techniques are only the tip of the iceberg. I did not describe many of the important theories regarding the complex interconnections these points have on the web of qi circulation. Those with comprehensive training in the acupuncture/acupressure system rely on these complex theories more than on what we considered in these chapters. If using these techniques is not effective for you, consult with a professional who specializes in acupuncture/acupressure.

CONCLUSION

The ancient Chinese left behind many mysteries, but none perhaps is more valuable to us today than their traditional medical system. As rapidly as acupuncture and other aspects of Chinese medicine are spreading throughout the world today, this system of health care is still being tragically undervalued and underused. I believe there are several reasons for this, some of which I have tried to address in this book: the lack of an accurate history of Chinese medicine's earliest roots, the seemingly subtle but actually critical difference between the Eastern and Western viewpoint on the role of spirituality in science, and the fact that there are two primary approaches to healing—what I have labeled action and reaction medicine.

In addition to these reasons, there are others I did not mention that I would like to briefly touch on here. One is related to the fact that modern medicine has spawned vast institutions such as hospitals, medical universities, the pharmaceutical industry, governmental oversight agencies, medical societies, the insurance industry, and so forth. Each of these institutions are run by a collection of individuals who have spent their entire professional careers dedicating themselves to learning all they could about their respective fields and working their way up the ladder into positions of authority. The average person might think that if something like acupuncture were to come along— something safe, effective, and extremely low-cost—those people in positions of authority would rush to include it into a medical system so tragically burdened with skyrocketing cost. Yet—the opposite has happened. Acupuncture and other forms of "alternative" care have been resisted and literally fought by the very people who, one would think, would be falling all over themselves to incorporate them into the mainstream. Why? In my opinion it is really quite simple: the leadership of these institutions feels their authority is threatened by

THE HEALING POWER OF ACUPRESSURE AND ACUPUNCTURE

these alternative approaches because they developed outside of these institutions and thus they know very little about them.

Chinese medicine especially represents such a threat because it not only comes from a different culture but also comes from the distant past, a past we were supposed to have left behind us as progress marched forward. For an authority in the modern medical field, such as those running these institutions, to acknowledge that Chinese medicine offers things of equal or, in some cases, even greater value than that of modern medicine, he would in essence be admitting that he is not the all-knowing authority his reputation suggests. In most cases this "threat to my authority" resistance is most likely subconscious; I doubt these individuals spend any time thinking to themselves that they had better fight the acceptance of these practices within their institutions because admitting they are legitimate will "make me look stupid." But for decision-makers to admit that something they know nothing about is of real value to their institution is understandably a difficult thing to do.

Frankly, I don't know if anything can be done about this institutional resistance; I guess it is just human nature. But I want to at least mention it, both in the hope that the general public can be made aware that this resistance is in part to blame for the failure of these institutions to do their job of looking out for useful new developments and also on the off chance that some individuals in positions of authority might read my thoughts and ask themselves if they have fallen prey to this all-too-human tendency.

Another factor that has kept Chinese medicine and other legitimate alternative approaches from being more appreciated is somewhat related to what I just described. In addition to undervaluing the strengths of alternative approaches, we have underestimated the weakness of the conventional (modern) approach, especially the damage done by drug therapy. It has only been since the late 1990s that some have begun to look seriously at the tragically high rate of complications caused by modern medical intervention (action medicine) in general and drug therapy in particular.

Recent studies published in prominent medical journals have shown that drug complications and medical errors rank between the third and fourth leading causes of death in the United States!* As bad as these statistics are, common sense tells us they represent only the tip of the iceberg. We have no way of knowing how much damage modern medical approaches may truly cause, as proving complications less dramatic than death is a difficult thing to do. Whatever the true damage and costs, both in human and financial terms, we need to pay more attention to just how risky action medicine is. If we were more honest with ourselves about this issue, then we would be compelled to look more seriously for safer alternatives. But here again, the fear of self-incrimination is holding us back. Those involved with modern health care will understandably be the last ones who want to admit they are causing more harm than previously thought. In addition, they don't believe there are safer alternatives, for the many reasons I have already considered. They will therefore tend to wonder why we should bother studying the problems with modern medicine if we have nothing better to replace it with.

While it is a very good sign that some brave individuals have begun to shed light on the fallout that action medicine has been causing, resistance and denial is slowing progress. If only the powers that be would wake up to the fact that there are legitimate, safer alternatives, perhaps we could make real progress to improve our health care system.

The last obstacle I wish to mention that is slowing a true integration of the best of both action and reaction medicine is that of profes-

---

*See Barbara Starfield, "Is US Health Really the Best in the World?" *Journal of the American Medical Association* 284 (July 2000); Linda Kohn, Janet Corrigan, and Molla Donaldson, *To Err is Human* (Washington, D.C.: National Academy Press, 1999); and Jason Lazarou, Bruce Pomeranz, and Paul Corey, "Incidence of Adverse Drug Reactions in Hospitalized Patients; A Meta-analysis of Prospective Studies," *Journal of the American Medical Association* 279 (April 1998).

sional turf. In chapter 8, I gave advice on how to find a qualified practitioner. This should have been a fairly simple thing to do, but it was actually one of the most difficult parts of writing this book. The growing interest in acupuncture, especially, has spawned disagreement over just who should be allowed to provide this therapy and what their training should be. To say that there are disagreements among those who practice acupuncture is an understatement. It is quite sad, in my opinion, that the growth of a wonderful new (to the West) healing approach would end up causing turf battles among its supporters. If those who understand the great value this healing approach affords us were to find a way to put differences aside and concentrate instead on overcoming the obstacles to its greater acceptance, we would make much more progress in getting this help to the people in need.

Because of the factors I have just described, my years of practicing Chinese medicine have been somewhat bittersweet for me. While I feel very fortunate to have learned about this important healing system and to have been able to help many people who were falling through the cracks of conventional care, it has also been frustrating knowing that so many more people could be helped if they only knew more about Chinese medicine. This book was born out of that frustration, and it is my hope that my efforts may make a small contribution toward a greater understanding of the treasure of healing possibilities that have stood the test of time and still await us, ready to serve us.

APPENDIX A

THE YELLOW EMPEROR'S TWELVE LAWS OF YIN AND YANG

From Hua-Ching Ni, *Tao: The Subtle Universal Law and the Integral Way of Life* (Los Angeles: Seven Star Communications, 1979).

1. That which produces and composes the universe is Tao, the undivided oneness or ultimate Nothingness.
2. Tao polarizes itself: yang becomes the active pole of the cosmos, yin becomes the solidified pole.
3. Yang and yin are opposites and each accomplishes the other.
4. All beings and things are complex aggregates of universal energy composed of infinitely varying proportions of yin and yang.
5. All beings and things are in a dynamic state of change; nothing is absolutely static or completed; all is in unceasing motion as polarization, the source of being, is without beginning and without end.

6. Yin and yang attract one another.

7. Nothing is entirely yin or entirely yang; all phenomena are composed of both yin and yang.

8. Nothing is neutral. All phenomena are composed of unequal proportions of yin and yang.

9. The force of attraction between yin and yang is greater when the difference between them is greater and smaller when it is smaller.

10. Like activities repel one another. The closer the similarity between two entities of the same polarity, the greater is their repulsion.

11. At the extremes of development, yin produces yang and yang produces yin.

12. All beings are yang in their essential core and yin in their physical makeup.

APPENDIX B

ANCIENT TAOIST

INSTRUCTIONS ON ATTAINING

THE ABSOLUTE MIND

Adaptation from Hsin Hsin Ming, translated by Seng-Tsan, active around 600 CE. From Hua-Ching Ni, *The Taoist Inner View of the Universe and the Immortal Realm* (Los Angeles: Seven Star Communications, 1979), pp. 152–6.

The integral Way is not difficult
   for those who have no preferences.
When love and hate are both absent
   the Way presents itself clearly.
Make the smallest distinction, however,
   and your distance from the truth is set apart like heaven and earth.
If you wish to recognize the truth,
   then hold no opinions for or against anything.

To set up what you like against what you dislike
  is the disease of the mind.

If the mind makes no discriminations,
  the ten thousand things are as they are, of single essence.
To understand the mystery of this one-essence
  is to be released from all entanglements.
When all things are seen equally,
  the timeless self-essence is reached.
No comparisons or analogies are possible
  in this causeless, relationless state.

For the complete instruction, please see Hua-Ching Ni's *The Taoist Inner View of the Universe and the Immortal Realm.*

RESOURCES

Resources for books on Chinese medicine and Taoist philosophy:

SevenStar Communications
13315 Washington Blvd., 2nd Floor
Los Angeles, CA 90066
1-310-302-1207, Fax: 1-310-302-1208
E-mail: taostar@taostar.com
www.sevenstar.com

Redwing Book Company
202 Bendix Drive
Taos, NM 87571
(800) 873-3946 Canada: (888) 873-3947
www.redwingbooks.com

Resources for finding qualified practitioners and other information regarding Chinese medicine:

National Certification Commission
   for Acupuncture and Oriental
   Medicine (NCCAOM)
11 Canal Center Plaza, Suite 300

Alexandria, VA 22314
(703) 548-9004
www.nccaom.org

American Association of Oriental
Medicine (AAOM)
909 22nd Street
Sacramento, CA 95816
(866) 455-7999
www.aaom.org

Acupuncture and Oriental Medicine
Alliance
6405 43rd Avenue Court NW, Suite B
Gig Harbor, WA 98335
(253) 851-6896
www.aomalliance.org

California State Oriental Medicine
Association (CSOMA)
P.O. Box 21246
Concord, CA 94521
(925) 687-8485

California Acupuncture Board
444 N. 3rd Street, Suite 260
Sacramento, CA 95814
(916) 445-3021

American Academy of Medical
Acupuncture Physicians (AAMA)
4929 Wilshire Blvd., Suite 428
Los Angeles, CA 90010-3817
(800) 521-2262
www.medicalacupuncture.org

Accrediting Commission for
Acupuncture and Oriental
Medicine (ACAOM)
Maryland Trade Center 3

7501 Greenway Center Drive, Suite 820
Greenbelt, MD 20770
(301) 313-0855
www.acaom.org

International Academy of Medical
Acupuncture (IAMA)
(800) 327-1113
www.IAMA.edu

Society for Acupuncture Research
www.acupunctureresearch.org

American Organization for
Bodywork Therapies of Asia
(AOBTA)
1010 Haddonfield-Berlin Road, Suite
408
Voorhees, NJ 08043-3514
(856) 782-1616
www.aobta.org

American Academy of Veterinary
Acupuncture (AAVA)
66 Morris Avenue, Suite 2A
Springfield, NJ 07081
(973) 379-1100
www.aava.org

BIBLIOGRAPHY

SOURCES ON ORIENTAL SCIENCE, HISTORY, AND CULTURE

Baskin, Wade. *Classics in Chinese Philosophy*. Totowa, NJ: Littlefield, Adams, 1974.

Beresford-Cooke, Carola. *Acupressure*. New York: Macmillan, 1996.

Campbell, Joseph. *The Masks of God: Oriental Mythology*. New York: Viking Penguin, 1962.

Campbell, Joseph. *The Masks of God: Primitive Mythology*. New York: Viking Press, 1959.

Ellis, Andrew, Nigel Wiseman, and Ken Boss. *Grasping the Wind*. Brookline, MA: Paradigm, 1989.

Fairservis, Walter A., Jr. *The Origins of Oriental Civilization*. New York: New American Library, 1959.

Gernet, Jacques. *A History of Chinese Civilization*. Translated by J. R. Foster. New York: Press Syndicate of the University of Cambridge, 1982.

Gongwang, Liu, and Akira Hyodo. *Fundamentals of Acupuncture and Moxibustion*. Tianjin, China: Tianjin Science and Technology, 1994.

Gwei-Djen, Ju, and Joseph Needham. *Celestial Lancets: A History and Rationale of Acupuncture and Moxa.* Cambridge, UK: Press Syndicate of the University of Cambridge, 1980.

Kaptchuk, Ted J. *The Web That Has No Weaver.* New York: Congdon and Weed, 1983.

Ni, Hua-Ching. *The Complete Works of Lao Tzu; Tao Teh Ching and Hua Hu Ching.* Los Angeles: Shrine of Eternal Breath of Tao, 1979.

Ni, Hua-Ching. *Eight Thousand Years of Wisdom: Conversations with Taoist Master Ni, Hua-Ching.* Los Angeles: Shrine of the Eternal Breath of Tao, 1983.

Ni, Hua-Ching. *Essence of Universal Spirituality.* Los Angeles: Shrine of the Eternal Breath of Tao, 1990.

Ni, Hua-Ching. *The Footsteps of the Mystical Child.* Los Angeles: Shrine of the Eternal Breath of Tao, 1986.

Ni, Hua-Ching. *The Gentle Path of Spiritual Progress.* Los Angeles: Shrine of the Eternal Breath of Tao, 1987.

Ni, Hua-Ching. *Guide to Inner Light.* Los Angeles: Shrine of the Eternal Breath of Tao, 1990.

Ni, Hua-Ching. *I Ching: The Book of Changes and the Unchanging Truth.* Los Angeles: Shrine of Eternal Breath of Tao, 1983.

Ni, Hua-Ching. *Tao: The Subtle Universal Law and the Integral Way of Life.* Los Angeles: Shrine of Eternal Breath of Tao, 1979.

Ni, Hua-Ching. *The Taoist Inner View of the Universe and the Immortal Realm.* Los Angeles: Seven Star Communications, 1979.

Ni, Hua-Ching. *Teachings of Chuang Tzu: Attaining Unlimited Life.* Los Angeles: Shrine of Eternal Breath of Tao, 1989.

Ni, Hua-Ching. *The Uncharted Voyage Toward The Subtle Light.* Los Angeles: Shrine of the Eternal Breath of Tao, 1985.

Ni, Hua-Ching. *Workbook for Spiritual Development of All People.* Los Angeles: Shrine of the Eternal Breath of Tao, 1984.

Ni, Maoshing, *The Yellow Emperor's Classic of Medicine.* Boston: Shambala, 1995.

Ohashi, Wataru. *Do-It-Yourself Shiatsu: How to Perform the Ancient Japanese Art of "Acupuncture without Needles."* New York: Dutton, 1976.

Palmer, Martin, ed. *T'ung Shu: The Ancient Chinese Almanac.* Boston: Shambala, 1986.

Porkert, Manfred. *The Essentials of Chinese Diagnostics.* Zurich: ACTA Medicinae Sinensis Chinese Medicine, 1983.

Spence, Jonathan D. *The Chan's Great Continent: China in Western Minds*. New York: Norton, 1998.

Temple, Robert. *The Genius of China: Three Thousand Years of Science, Discovery, and Invention*. New York: Simon and Schuster, 1989.

Time-Life Books. *TimeFrame 1500–600 BC: Barbarian Tides*. Alexandria, VA: Time-Life Books, 1987.

Time-Life Books. *TimeFrame 3000–1500 BC: The Age of God-Kings*. Alexandria, VA: Time-Life Books, 1987.

Unschuld, Paul U. *Chinese Medicine*. Brookline, MA: Paradigm, 1998.

Unschuld, Paul U. *Huang Di Nei Jing Su Wen: Nature, Knowledge, Imagery in an Ancient Chinese Medical Text*. Berkeley: University of California Press, 2003.

Unschuld, Paul U. *Medicine in China: A History of Ideas*. Berkeley: University of California Press, 1985.

Veith, Ilza. *The Yellow Emperor's Classic of Internal Medicine*. Berkeley: University of California, 1966.

Watson, William. *China: Before the Han Dynasty*. New York: Praeger, 1961.

Werner, Edward T. C. *Ancient Tales and Folklore of China*. London: Bracken Books, 1986.

Whittaker, Clio. *An Introduction to Oriental Mythology*. Secaucus, NJ: Chartwell Books, 1989.

Xin, Yang, Richard M. Barnhart, Nie Chongzheng, James Cahill, Lang Shaojun, and Wu Hung. *Three Thousand Years of Chinese Painting*. New Haven, CT: Foreign Languages Press, 1997.

SOURCES ON WESTERN SCIENCE, HISTORY, AND CULTURE

Bordley, James III and Harvey A. McGehee. *Two Centuries of American Medicine*. Philadelphia: Saunders, 1976.

Capra, Fritjof. *The Tao of Physics*. Boulder, CO: Shambala, 1983.

Capra, Fritjof. *The Web of Life: A New Scientific Understanding of Living Systems*. New York: Doubleday, 1996.

Chaisson, Eric. *Relatively Speaking: Relativity, Black Holes, and the Fate of the Universe*. New York: Norton, 1990.

Cho, Z. H., E. K. Wong, and J. Fallon. *Neuro-Acupuncture: Scientific evidence of Acupuncture Revealed*. Los Angeles: Q-puncture, 2001.

Cohen, Bernard I. *The Birth of a New Physics*. New York: Norton, 1960.

Coveney, Peter, and Roger Highfield. *The Arrow of Time.* New York: Ballantine Books, 1990.

Duncan, David Ewing. *Calendar: Humanity's Epic Struggle to Determine a True and Accurate Year.* New York: Avon Books, 1998.

Eisler, Riane. *The Chalice and the Blade: Our History, Our Future.* New York: HarperCollins, 1987.

Fisher, Jeffrey A. *The Plague Makers.* New York: Simon and Schuster, 1994.

Gleick, James. *Chaos: The Making of a New Science.* New York: Penguin Books, 1987.

Hawking, Stephen. *A Brief History of Time: From the Big Bang to Black Holes.* New York: Bantam Books, 1988.

Krupp, E. C. *Beyond the Blue Horizon: Myths and Legends of the Sun, Moon, Stars, and Planets.* New York: HarperCollins, 1991.

Motz, Lloyd. *The Constellations.* New York: Doubleday, 1988.

Prigogine, Ilya, and Isabelle Stengers. *Order Out of Chaos: Man's New Dialogue with Nature.* New York: Bantam Books, 1984.

Schick, Kathy D., and Nicholas Toth. *Making Silent Stones Speak.* New York: Simon and Schuster, 1993.

Sherman I. W. and V. G. Sherman. *Biology: A Human Approach.* 3rd ed. New York: Oxford University Press, 1983.

Starr, Paul. *The Social Transformation of American Medicine.* New York: Basic Books, 1982.

INDEX

ABOUT THE AUTHOR

Matthew D. Bauer L.Ac., became interested in Eastern philosophy as a teenager as a result of his interest in the martial arts. When a serious back injury at age seventeen failed to respond to conventional care, he eventually came to study acupressure. At age twenty-two, he met and became a student of a leading world authority on the subject of Taoism—a seventy-fourth generation Taoist master named Hua-Ching Ni. This began what would turn into a lifelong study of Taoist philosophy, folk history, and spirituality, as well as the study and practice of acupuncture and Chinese medicine.

After becoming involved with acupuncture professional associations in the late 1980s, Matthew developed a passion for educating the public about the benefits of acupuncture, acupressure, and Chinese medicine, especially the roots of this ancient healing system.

Matthew resides in La Verne, California, with his wife, Gayle, and dog, Cleo, and has two grown sons who live nearby. Matthew maintains a full-time healing practice at La Verne Acupuncture. He can be contacted through his website, www.MatthewDBauer.com.

Stuart Woods - Stone Barrington
series

David Baldacci - w/ "Saving Faith"

Michael Connally   Harry Bosch
                          series
                          "Black Echo"
Robert Parker -   Jessie
Brad Metzger -   Stone series
                          First Council
James   Patterson   Alex Cross
                              series

Lodging   1,000
Fishing   200
Sanitary   130
Lunch Amtk   55
Aquarium   45
Lunch Basket   30
Bus Tour   30
Gas   150 — 1660
Raleigh Hotel ≈ 400 (?) 785
                        $2445

Coldstone   30
Lunch Sat   25
BBQ   Mon   50
Lunch Mon   30
Dinner Sun   55
Lunch Sun   30
Lunch Tues   25
Lunch Wed   20
Tues Dinner   120